Virtual Clinical Excursions—General Hospital

for

Potter and Perry:
Basic Nursing,
6th Edition

Virtual Clinical Excursions—General Hospital

for

Potter and Perry:
Basic Nursing,
6th Edition

prepared by

Patricia A. Potter, RN, MSN, PhD, CMAC, FAAN
Research Scientist
Barnes-Jewish Hospital
St. Louis, Missouri

Amy Hall, RN, BSN, MS, PhD
Associate Professor
Saint Francis Medical Center College of Nursing
Peoria, Illinois

software developed by

Wolfsong Informatics, LLC
Tucson, Arizona

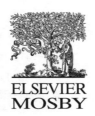

ELSEVIER
MOSBY

ELSEVIER
MOSBY

11830 Westline Industrial Dr.
St. Louis, Missouri 63146

VIRTUAL CLINICAL EXCURSIONS—GENERAL HOSPITAL FOR
POTTER AND PERRY: BASIC NURSING,
SIXTH EDITION

ISBN-13: 978-0-323-04616-9
ISBN-10: 0-323-04616-9

Copyright © 2007 by Mosby, Inc., an affiliate of Elsevier Inc.

Notice

Knowledge and best practice in this field are constantly changing. As new research and experience broaden our knowledge, changes in practice, treatment and drug therapy may become necessary or appropriate. Readers are advised to check the most current information provided (i) on procedures featured or (ii) by the manufacturer of each product to be administered, to verify the recommended dose or formula, the method and duration of administration, and contraindications. It is the responsibility of the practitioner, relying on their own experience and knowledge of the patient, to make diagnoses, to determine dosages and the best treatment for each individual patient, and to take all appropriate safety precautions. To the fullest extent of the law, neither the Publisher nor the Authors assumes any liability for any injury and/or damage to persons or property arising out or related to any use of the material contained in this book.

ISBN-13: 978-0-323-04616-9
ISBN-10: 0-323-04616-9

Executive Editor: *Tom Wilhelm*
Managing Editor: *Jeff Downing*
Associate Developmental Editor: *Tiffany Pfaff*
Project Manager: *Joy Moore*

Printed in the United States of America

Last digit is the print number: 9 8 7 6 5 4 3 2 1

*Workbook
prepared by*

Patricia A. Potter, RN, MSN, PhD, CMAC, FAAN
Research Scientist
Barnes-Jewish Hospital
St. Louis, Missouri

Amy Hall, RN, BSN, MS, PhD
Associate Professor
Saint Francis Medical Center College of Nursing
Peoria, Illinois

Textbook

Patricia A. Potter, RN, MSN, PhD, CMAC, FAAN
Research Scientist
Barnes-Jewish Hospital
St. Louis, Missouri

Anne Griffin Perry, RN, MSN, EdD, FAAN
Chair
Department of Primary Care and Health Systems Nursing
Southern Illinois University
Edwardsville, Illinois

Contents

Table of Contents
Potter and Perry
Basic Nursing, 6th Edition

Getting Started

GETTING SET UP

■ MINIMUM SYSTEM REQUIREMENTS

WINDOWS™

Windows XP, 2000, 98, ME, NT 4.0 (Recommend Windows XP/2000)
Pentium® III processor (or equivalent) @ 600 MHz (Recommend 800 MHz or better)
128 MB of RAM (Recommend 256 MB or more)
800 x 600 screen size (Recommend 1024 x 768)
Thousands of colors
12x CD-ROM drive
Soundblaster 16 soundcard compatibility
Stereo speakers or headphones

Note: Virtual Clinical Excursions—General Hospital for Windows will require a minimal amount of disk space to install icons and required dll files for Windows 98/ME.

MACINTOSH®

MAC OS X (10.2 or higher)
Apple Power PC G3 @ 500 MHz or better
128 MB of RAM (Recommend 256 MB or more)
800 x 600 screen size (Recommend 1024 x 768)
Thousands of colors
12x CD-ROM drive
Stereo speakers or headphones

■ INSTALLATION INSTRUCTIONS

WINDOWS

1. Insert the *Virtual Clinical Excursions—General Hospital* CD-ROM.
2. Inserting the CD should automatically bring up the setup screen if the current product is not already installed.
   a. If the setup screen does not appear automatically (and *Virtual Clinical Excursions—General Hospital* has not been installed already), navigate to the "My Computer" icon on your desktop or in your Start menu.
   b. Double-click on your CD-ROM drive.
   c. If installation does not start at this point:
      (1) Click the **Start** icon on the task bar and select the **Run** option.
      (2) Type d:\setup.exe (where "d:\" is your CD-ROM drive) and press **OK**.
      (3) Follow the onscreen instructions for installation.
3. Follow the onscreen instructions during the setup process.

MACINTOSH

1. Insert the *Virtual Clinical Excursions—General Hospital* CD in the CD-ROM drive. The disk icon will appear on your desktop.

2. Double-click on the disk icon.

3. Double-click on the GENERAL-HOSPITAL_MAC run file.

NOTE: *Virtual Clinical Excursions—General Hospital* for Macintosh does not have an installation setup and can only be run directly from the CD.

■ HOW TO USE VIRTUAL CLINICAL EXCURSIONS—GENERAL HOSPITAL

WINDOWS

1. Double-click on the *Virtual Clinical Excursions—General Hospital* icon located on your desktop.
2. Or navigate to the program via the Windows Start menu.

NOTE: Windows 98/ME will require you to restart your computer before running the *Virtual Clinical Excursions—General Hospital* program.

MACINTOSH

1. Insert the *Virtual Clinical Excursions—General Hospital* CD in the CD-ROM drive. The disk icon will appear on your desktop.

2. Double-click on the disk icon.

3. Double-click on the GENERAL-HOSPITAL_MAC run file.

■ SCREEN SETTINGS

For best results, your computer monitor resolution should be set at a minimum of 800 x 600. The number of colors displayed should be set to "thousands or higher" (High Color or 16 bit) or "millions of colors" (True Color or 24 bit).

Windows™

1. From the **Start** menu, select **Control Panel** (on some systems, you will first go to **Settings**, then to **Control Panel**).
2. Double-click on the **Display** icon.
3. Click on the **Settings** tab.
4. Under **Screen area** use the slider bar to select **800 by 600 pixels**.
5. Access the **Colors** drop-down menu by clicking on the down arrow.
6. Select **High Color (16 bit)** or **True Color (24 bit)**.
7. Click on **OK**.
8. You may be asked to verify the setting changes. Click **Yes**.
9. You may be asked to restart your computer to accept the changes. Click **Yes**.

Macintosh®

1. Select the **Monitors** control panel.
2. Select **800 x 600** (or similar) from the **Resolution** area.
3. Select **Thousands** or **Millions** from the **Color Depth** area.

■ WEB BROWSERS

Supported web browsers include Microsoft Internet Explorer (IE) version 6.0 or higher, Netscape version 7.1 or higher, and Mozilla version 1.4 or higher.

If you use America Online (AOL) for web access, you will need AOL version 4.0 or higher and IE 5.0 or higher. Do not use earlier versions of AOL with earlier versions of IE, because you will have difficulty accessing many features.

For best results with AOL:
- Connect to the Internet using AOL version 4.0 or higher.
- Open a private chat within AOL (this allows the AOL client to remain open, without asking whether you wish to disconnect while minimized).
- Minimize AOL.
- Launch a recommended browser.

■ TECHNICAL SUPPORT

Technical support for this product is available between 7:30 a.m. and 7 p.m. CST, Monday through Friday. Before calling, be sure that your computer meets the minimum system requirements to run this software. Inside the United States and Canada, call 1-800-692-9010. Outside North America, call 314-872-8370. You may also fax your questions to 314-523-4932 or contact Technical Support through e-mail: technical.support@elsevier.com.

Trademarks: Windows, Macintosh, Pentium, and America Online are registered trademarks.

Copyright © 2007 by Mosby, Inc., an affiliate of Elsevier Inc.

ACCESSING *Virtual Clinical Excursions—General-Hospital* FROM EVOLVE

The product you have purchased is part of the Evolve family of online courses and learning resources. Please read the following information completely to get started.

To access your instructor's course on Evolve:

Your instructor will provide you with the username and password needed to access their specific course on the Evolve Learning System. Once you have received this information, please follow these instructions:

1. Go to the Evolve student page (http://evolve.elsevier.com/student)

2. Enter your username and password in the **Login to My Evolve** area and click the **Login** button.

3. You will be taken to your personalized **My Evolve** page where the course will be listed in the **My Courses** module.

TECHNICAL REQUIREMENTS

To use an Evolve course, you will need access to a computer that is connected to the Internet and equipped with web browser software that supports frames. For optimal performance, it is recommended that you have speakers and use a high-speed Internet connection. However, slower dial-up modems (56 K minimum) are acceptable.

Whichever browser you use, the browser preferences must be set to enable cookies and Java/JavaScript and the cache must be set to reload every time.

Enable Cookies

Browser	Steps
Internet Explorer (IE) 6.0 or higher	1. Select **Tools**. 2. Select **Internet Options**. 3. Select **Privacy** tab. 4. Use the slider (slide down) to **Accept All Cookies**. 5. Click **OK**. -OR- 4. Click the **Advanced** button. 5. Click the check box next to **Override Automatic Cookie Handling**. 6. Click the **Accept** buttons under **First-party Cookies** and **Third-party Cookies**. 7. Click **OK**.
Netscape 7.1 or higher	1. Select **Edit**. 2. Select **Preferences**. 3. Select **Privacy & Security**. 4. Select **Cookies**. 5. Select **Enable All Cookies**.
Mozilla 1.4 or higher	1. Select **Tools**. 2. Select **Privacy**. 3. Expand the **Cookies** section and check the following box: Allow sites to set cookies.

Enable Java

Browser	Steps
Internet Explorer (IE) 6.0 or higher	1. Select **Tools → Internet Options**. 2. Select **Advanced** tab. 3. Scroll down the list until you see the **Java (Sun)** section and select the box that appears below it.
Netscape 7.1 or higher	1. Select **Edit → Preferences**. 2. Select **Advanced**. 3. Select **Scripts & Plugins**. 4. Make sure the **Navigator** box is checked to **Enable JavaScript**. 5. Click **OK**.
Mozilla 1.4 or higher	1. Select **Tools**. 2. Select **Web Features**. 3. Select the boxes next to **Enable Java** and **Enable JavaScript**.

Set Cache to Always Reload a Page

Browser	Steps
Internet Explorer (IE) 6.0 or higher	1. Select **Tools → Internet Options**. 2. Select **General** tab. 3. Go to the **Temporary Internet Files** and click the **Settings** button. 4. Select the radio button for **Every visit to the page** and click **OK** when complete.
Netscape 7.1 or higher	1. Select **Edit → Preferences**. 2. Select **Advanced**. 3. Select **Cache**. 4. Select the **Every time I view the page** radio button. 5. Click **OK**.
Mozilla 1.4 or higher	1. Select **Tools**. 2. Select **Privacy**. 3. Expand the **Cache** section and designate a disk space number if one isn't in place already.

Plug-Ins

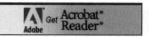

Adobe Acrobat Reader—With the free Acrobat Reader software you can view and print Adobe PDF files. Many Evolve products offer student and instructor manuals, checklists, and more in this format!

Download at: *http://www.adobe.com*

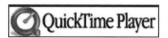

Apple QuickTime—Install this to hear word pronunciations, heart and lung sounds, and many other helpful audio clips within Evolve Online Courses!

Download at: *http://www.apple.com*

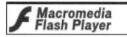

Macromedia Flash Player—This player will enhance your viewing of many Evolve web pages, as well as educational short-form to long-form animation within the Evolve Learning System!

Download at: *http://www.macromedia.com*

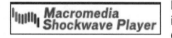

Macromedia Shockwave Player—Shockwave is best for viewing the many interactive learning activities within Evolve Online Courses!

Download at: *http://www.macromedia.com*

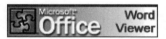

Microsoft Word Viewer—With this viewer Microsoft Word users can share documents with those who don't have Word, and users without Word can open and view Word documents. Many Evolve products have testbank, student and instructor manuals, and other documents available for downloading and viewing on your own computer!

Download at: *http://www.microsoft.com*

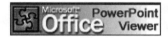

Microsoft PowerPoint Viewer—View PowerPoint 97, 2000, and 2002 presentations even if you don't have PowerPoint with this viewer. Many Evolve products have slides available for downloading and viewing on your own computer!

Download at: *http://www.microsoft.com*

SUPPORT INFORMATION

Live support is available to customers in the United States and Canada from 7:30 a.m. to 7:00 p.m. (Central Time), Monday through Friday by calling, **1-800-401-9962**. You can also send an email to evolve-support@elsevier.com.

There is also **24/7 support information** available on the Evolve website (http://evolve.elsevier.com), including:

- Guided Tours
- Tutorials
- Frequently Asked Questions (FAQs)
- Online Copies of Course User Guides
- And much more!

A QUICK TOUR

Welcome to *Virtual Clinical Excursions—General Hospital*, a virtual hospital setting in which you can work with multiple complex patient simulations and also learn to access and evaluate the information resources that are essential for high-quality patient care.

The virtual hospital, Pacific View Regional Hospital, has realistic architecture and access to patient rooms, a Nurses' Station, and a Medication Room.

■ BEFORE YOU START

Make sure you have your textbook nearby when you use the *Virtual Clinical Excursions— General Hospital* CD. You will want to consult topic areas in your textbook frequently while working with the CD and using this workbook.

■ HOW TO SIGN IN

- Enter your name on the Student Nurse identification badge.
- Now click the down arrow next to **Select Period of Care**. This drop-down menu gives you four periods of care from which to choose. In Periods of Care 1 through 3, you can actively engage in patient assessment, entry of data in the electronic patient record (EPR), and medication administration. Period of Care 4 presents the day in review. Highlight and click the appropriate period of care. (For this quick tour, choose **Period of Care 2**.)
- Click **Go** in the lower right side of the screen.
- This takes you to the Patient List screen (see example on page 11). Only the patients on the floor you choose (e.g., Medical-Surgical) are available. Note that the virtual time is provided in the box at the lower left corner of the screen (1115, since we chose Period of Care 2).

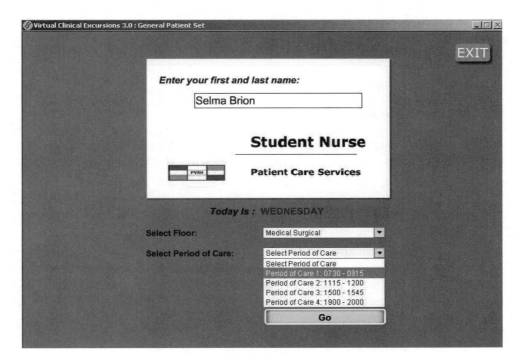

■ **PATIENT LIST**

MEDICAL-SURGICAL UNIT

Harry George (Room 401)
Osteomyelitis—A middle-aged Caucasian male admitted from a homeless shelter with an infected leg. He has complications of type 2 diabetes mellitus, alcohol abuse, nicotine addiction, poor pain control, and complex psychosocial issues.

Jacquline Catanazaro (Room 402)
Asthma—A middle-aged Caucasian female admitted with an acute asthma exacerbation and suspected pneumonia. She has complications of chronic schizophrenia, noncompliance with medication therapy, obesity, and herniated disc.

Piya Jordan (Room 403)
Bowel obstruction—An older Asian female admitted with a colon mass and suspected adenocarcinoma. She undergoes a right hemicolectomy. This patient's complications include atrial fibrillation, hypokalemia, and symptoms of meperidine toxicity.

Clarence Hughes (Room 404)
Degenerative joint disease—An older African-American male admitted for a left total knee replacement. His preparations for discharge are complicated by the development of a pulmonary embolus and the need for ongoing intravenous therapy.

Pablo Rodriguez (Room 405)
Metastatic lung carcinoma—An older Hispanic male admitted with symptoms of dehydration and malnutrition. He has chronic pain secondary to multiple subcutaneous skin nodules and psychosocial concerns related to family issues with his approaching death.

Patricia Newman (Room 406)
Pneumonia—A middle-aged Caucasian female admitted with worsening pulmonary function and an acute respiratory infection. Her chronic emphysema is complicated by heavy smoking, hypertension, and malnutrition. She needs access to community resources such as a smoking cessation program and meal assistance.

SKILLED NURSING UNIT

William Jefferson (Room 501)
Alzheimer's disease—An elderly African-American male admitted for stabilization of type 2 diabetes and hypertension following a recent acute care admission for a urinary tract infection and sepsis. His complications include episodes of acute delirium and a history of osteoarthritis.

Kathryn Doyle (Room 503)
Rehabilitation post left hip replacement—An elderly Caucasian female admitted following a complicated recovery from an ORIF. She is experiencing symptoms of malnutrition and depression due to unstable family dynamics, placing her at risk for elder abuse.

Goro Oishi (Room 505)
Hospice care—An older Asian male admitted following an acute care admission for an intracerebral hemorrhage and resulting coma. Family-staff interactions provide opportunities to explore death and dying issues related to conflict about advanced life support and cultural and religious differences.

OBSTETRICS UNIT

Dorothy Grant (Room 201)
30-week intrauterine pregnancy—A young multipara admitted with abdominal trauma following a domestic violence incident. Her complications include preterm labor and extensive social issues such as acquiring safe housing for her family upon discharge.

■ HOW TO SELECT A PATIENT

- You can choose one or more patients to work with from the Patient List by clicking the box to the left of the patient name(s). (In order to receive a scorecard for a patient, the patient must be selected before proceeding to the Nurses' Station.)
- Click on **Get Report** to the right of the medical records number (MRN) to view a summary of the patient's care during the 12-hour period before your arrival on the unit.
- After reviewing the report, click on **Return to Patient List**.
- When you are ready to begin your care, click on **Go to Nurses' Station** in the right lower corner.

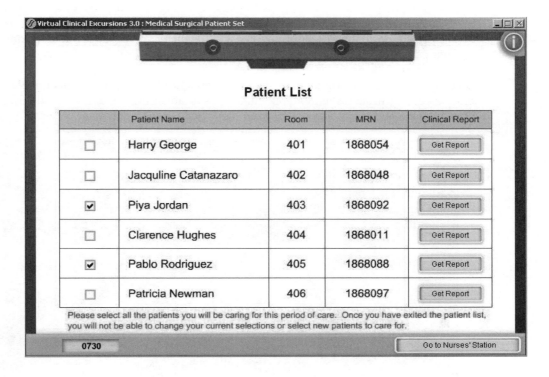

Virtual Clinical Excursions 3.0 : Medical Surgical Patient Set

Patient List

	Patient Name	Room	MRN	Clinical Report
☐	Harry George	401	1868054	Get Report
☐	Jacquline Catanazaro	402	1868048	Get Report
☑	Piya Jordan	403	1868092	Get Report
☐	Clarence Hughes	404	1868011	Get Report
☑	Pablo Rodriguez	405	1868088	Get Report
☐	Patricia Newman	406	1868097	Get Report

Please select all the patients you will be caring for this period of care. Once you have exited the patient list, you will not be able to change your current selections or select new patients to care for.

0730

Go to Nurses' Station

■ HOW TO FIND A PATIENT'S RECORDS

NURSES' STATION

Within the Nurses' Station, you will see:

1. A clipboard that contains the patient list for that floor.
2. A chart rack with patient charts labeled by room number, a notebook labeled Kardex, and a notebook labeled MAR (Medication Administration Record).
3. A desktop computer with access to the Electronic Patient Record (EPR).
4. A tool bar across the top of the screen that can also be used to access the Patient List, EPR, Chart, MAR, and Kardex. This tool bar is also accessible from each patient's room.
5. A Drug Guide containing information about the medications you are able to administer to your patients.

As you run your cursor over an item, it will be highlighted. To select, simply double-click on the item. As you use these resources, you will always be able to return to the Nurses' Station by clicking on the **Return to Nurses' Station** bar located in the right lower corner of your screen.

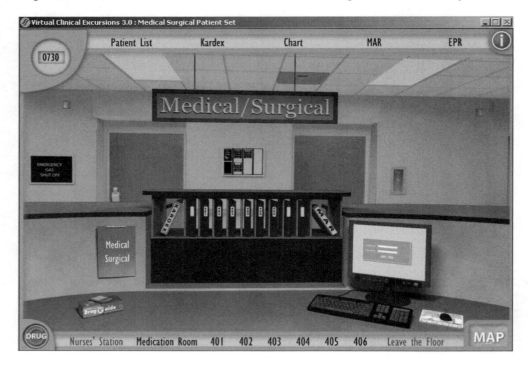

MEDICATION ADMINISTRATION RECORD (MAR)

The MAR icon located in the tool bar at the top of your screen accesses current 24-hour medications for each patient. Click on the icon and the MAR will open. (*Note:* You can also access the MAR by clicking on the blue MAR notebook on the far right side of the book rack in the center of the screen.) Within the MAR, tabs on the right side of the screen allow you to select patients by room number. Be careful to make sure you select the correct tab number for *your* patient rather than simply reading the first record that appears after the MAR opens. Each MAR sheet lists the following:

- Medications
- Route and dosage of medications
- Times of administration of medication

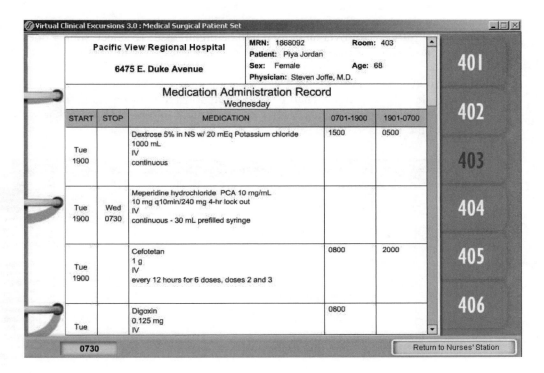

Note: The MAR changes each day. Expired MARs are stored in the patients' charts.

CHARTS

To access patient charts, either click on the **Chart** icon at the top of your screen or anywhere within the chart rack in the center of the Nurses' Station screen. When the close-up view appears, the individual charts are labeled by room number. To open a chart, click on the room number of the patient whose chart you wish to review. The patient's name and allergies will appear, along with a list of tabs on the right side of the screen, allowing you to view the following data:

- Allergies
- Physician's Orders
- Physician's Notes
- Nurse's Notes
- Laboratory Reports
- Diagnostic Reports
- Surgical Reports
- Consultations

- Patient Education
- History and Physical
- Nursing Admission
- Expired MARs
- Consents
- Mental Health
- Admissions
- Emergency Department

Information appears in real time. The entries are in reverse chronological order, so use the down arrow at the right side of the chart page to scroll down to view previous entries. Flip from tab to tab to view multiple data fields or click on the **Return to Nurses' Station** bar in the lower right corner of the screen to exit the chart.

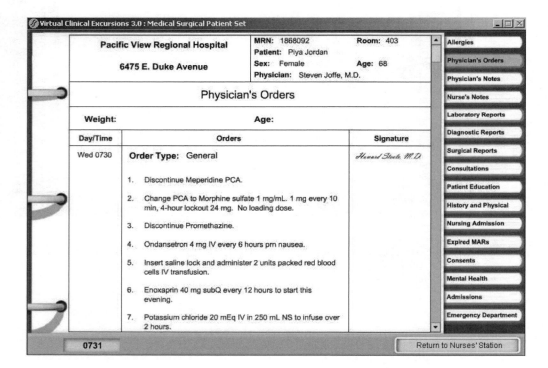

ELECTRONIC PATIENT RECORD (EPR)

The EPR can be accessed from the computer in the Nurses' Station or from the EPR icon located in the tool bar at the top of your screen. To access a patient's EPR:
- Click on either the computer screen or the **EPR** icon.
- Your user name and password are automatically filled in.
- Click on **Login** to enter the EPR.

The EPR used in Pacific View Regional Hospital represents a composite of commercial versions being used in hospitals. You can access the EPR:
- for a patient (by room number).
- to review existing data.
- to enter data you collect while working with a patient.

The EPR is updated daily, so no matter what day or part of a shift you are working, there will be a current EPR with the patient's data from the past days of the current hospital stay. This type of simulated EPR allows you to examine how data for different attributes have changed over time, as well as to examine data for all of a patient's attributes at a particular time. The EPR is fully functional (as it is in a real-life hospital). You can enter such data as blood pressure, breath sounds, and certain treatments. The EPR will not, however, allow you to enter data for a previous time period. Use the arrows at the bottom of the screen to move forward and backward in time.

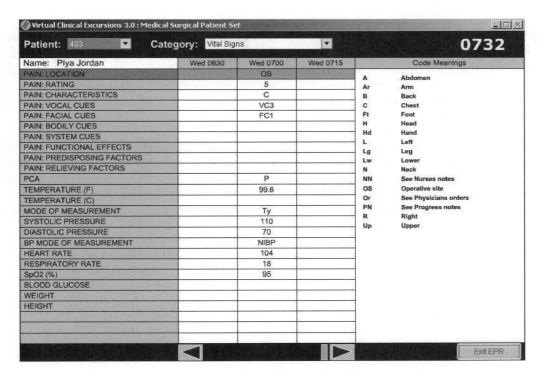

Name: Piya Jordan	Wed 0630	Wed 0700	Wed 0715	Code Meanings	
PAIN: LOCATION		OS		A	Abdomen
PAIN: RATING		5		Ar	Arm
PAIN: CHARACTERISTICS		C		B	Back
PAIN: VOCAL CUES		VC3		C	Chest
PAIN: FACIAL CUES		FC1		Ft	Foot
PAIN: BODILY CUES				H	Head
PAIN: SYSTEM CUES				Hd	Hand
PAIN: FUNCTIONAL EFFECTS				L	Left
PAIN: PREDISPOSING FACTORS				Lg	Leg
PAIN: RELIEVING FACTORS				Lw	Lower
PCA		P		N	Neck
TEMPERATURE (F)		99.6		NN	See Nurses notes
TEMPERATURE (C)				OS	Operative site
MODE OF MEASUREMENT		Ty		Or	See Physicians orders
SYSTOLIC PRESSURE		110		PN	See Progress notes
DIASTOLIC PRESSURE		70		R	Right
BP MODE OF MEASUREMENT		NIBP		Up	Upper
HEART RATE		104			
RESPIRATORY RATE		18			
SpO2 (%)		95			
BLOOD GLUCOSE					
WEIGHT					
HEIGHT					

Patient: 403   Category: Vital Signs   0732

At the top of the EPR screen, you can choose patients by their room numbers. In addition, you have access to 17 different categories of patient data. To change patients or data categories, click the down arrow to the right of the room number or category.

The categories of patient data in the EPR as as follows:

- Vital Signs
- Respiratory
- Cardiovascular
- Neurologic
- Gastrointestinal
- Excretory
- Musculoskeletal
- Integumentary
- Reproductive
- Psychosocial
- Wounds and Drains
- Activity
- Hygiene and Comfort
- Safety
- Nutrition
- IV
- Intake and Output

Remember, each hospital selects its own codes. The codes used in the EPR at Pacific View Regional Hospital may be different from ones you have seen in clinical rotations that have computerized patient records. Take some time to acquaint yourself with the codes. Within the Vital Signs category, click on any item in the left column (e.g., heart rate). In the far-right column, you will see a list of code meanings for the possible findings and/or descriptors for that assessment area.

You will use the codes to record the data you collect as you work with patients. Click on the box in the last time column to the right of the data and wait for the code meanings applicable to that entry to appear. Select the appropriate code to describe your assessment findings and type it in the box. (*Note:* If no cursor appears within the box, click on the box again until the blue shading disappears and the blinking cursor appears.) Once the data are typed in this box, they are entered into the patient's record for this period of care only.

To leave the EPR, click on **Exit EPR** in the bottom right corner of the screen.

■ **VISITING A PATIENT**

From the Nurses' Station, click on the room number of the patient you wish to visit in the tool bar at the bottom of your screen. Once you are inside the room, you will see a still photo of your patient in the top left corner. To verify that this is the patient you have chosen, click on the **Check Armband** icon to the right of the photo. The patient's identification data will appear. If you click on **Check Allergies** (the next icon to the right), a list of the patient's allergies (if any) will replace the photo.

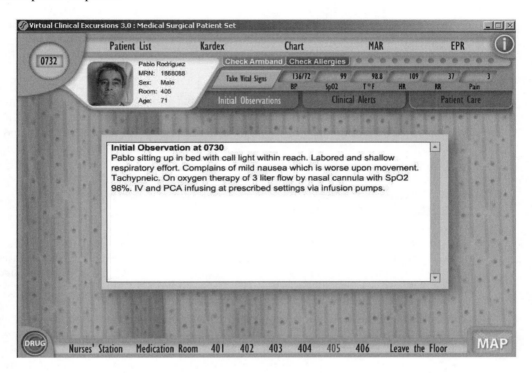

Also located in the patient's room are multiple icons you may use to assess the patient or the patient's medications. A clock is provided in the upper left corner of the room to monitor your progress in real time.

- The tool bar across the top of the screen allows you to check the **Patient List**, access the **EPR** to check or enter data, and view the patient's **Chart**, **MAR**, or **Kardex**.

- The **Take Vital Signs** icon allows you to measure the patient's up-to-the-minute blood pressure, oxygen saturation, temperature, heart rate, respiratory rate, and pain level.

- When you click on **Initial Observations**, a description appears in the text box under the patient's photo, allowing you a "look" at the patient as if you had just stepped in. To the right of this icon is **Clinical Alerts**, a resource that allows you to make decisions about priority medication interventions based on emerging data collected in real time. Check this screen throughout your period of care to avoid missing critical information related to recently ordered or STAT medications.

- Clicking on the **Patient Care** icon opens up three specific learning environments within the patient room: **Physical Assessment**, **Nurse-Client Interactions**, and **Medication Administration**.

- To perform a **Physical Assessment**, choose a body area (such as **Head & Neck**) by clicking on the appropriate icon in the column of yellow buttons. This activates a list of system subcategories for that body area (e.g., see **Sensory**, **Neurologic**, etc. in the green boxes). After you click on the system that you wish to evaluate, a still photo and text box appear, describing the assessment findings. The still photo is a "snapshot" of how an assessment of this area might be done or what the finding might look like. For every body area, there is also an **Equipment** button located on the far right of the screen.

- To the right of the Physical Assessment icon is **Nurse-Client Interactions**. Clicking on this icon will reveal the times and titles of any videos available for viewing. (*Note:* If the video you wish to see is not listed, this means you have not yet reached the correct virtual time to view that video. Check the virtual clock; you may return to access the video once its designated time has occurred—as long as you do so within the corresponding period of care.) To view a listed video, click on the white arrow to the right of the video title. Use the square control buttons below the video to start, stop, pause, rewind, or fast-forward the action or to mute the sound.

- **Medication Administration** is the pathway that allows you to review and administer medications to a patient after you have prepared them in the Medication Room. This process is addressed further in the *How to Prepare Medications* section (pages 19-20) and in *Medications* (pages 26-30). For additional hands-on practice, see *Reducing Medication Errors* (pages 37-41).

■ HOW TO QUIT, CHANGE PATIENTS, CHANGE FLOORS, OR CHANGE PERIOD OF CARE

How to Quit: From most screens, you may click the **Leave the Floor** icon on the bottom tool bar to the right of the patient room numbers. (*Note:* From some screens, you will first need to click an **Exit** button or **Return to Nurses' Station** before clicking **Leave the Floor**.) When the Floor Menu appears, click **Exit** to leave the program.

How to Change Patients, Floors, or Period of Care: To change patients, simply click on the new patient's room number. (You cannot receive a scorecard for a new patient, however, unless you have already selected that patient on the Patient List screen.) To change to a new period of care, to change floors, or to restart the virtual clock for a new patient, click on **Leave the Floor** and then on **Restart the Program**.

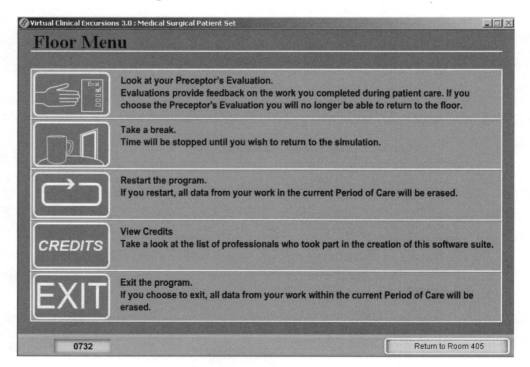

■ HOW TO PREPARE MEDICATIONS

From the Nurses' Station or the patient's room, you can access the Medication Room by clicking on the icon in the tool bar at the bottom of your screen to the left of the patient room numbers.

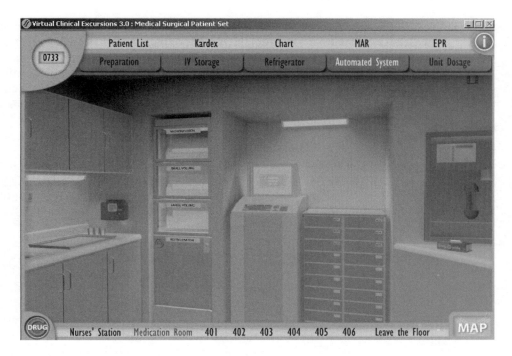

In the Medication Room you have access to the following (from left to right):

- A preparation area is located on the counter under the cabinets. To begin the medication preparation process, click on the tray on the counter or click on the **Preparation** icon at the top of the screen. The next screen leads you through a preparation sequence (called the Preparation Wizard) to prepare medications one at a time for administration to a patient. However, no medication has been selected at this time. We will do this while working with a patient in *A Detailed Tour*. To exit this screen, click on **View the Medication Room**.

- To the right of the cabinets (and above the refrigerator), IV storage bins are provided. Click on the bins themselves or on the **IV Storage** icon at the top of the screen. The bins are labeled **Microinfusion**, **Small Volume**, and **Large Volume**. Click on an individual bin to see a list of its contents. No medications are available in the bins at this time, but if they were, you could click on an individual medication and its label would appear to the right under the patient's name. Next, you would click **Put Medication on Tray**. If you ever change your mind or choose the incorrect medication, you can reverse your actions by clicking on **Put Medication in Bin**. Click **Close Bin** in the right bottom corner to exit. **View Medication Room** brings you back to a full view of the entire room.

- A refrigerator is located under the IV storage bins to hold any medications that must be stored below room temperature. Click on it to remove your medications; then click **Close Door**. You can also access this area by clicking the **Refrigerator** icon at the top of the screen.

- To prepare controlled substances, click the **Automated System** icon at the top of the screen or click the computer monitor located to the right of the IV storage bins. A login screen will appear; your name and password are automatically filled in. Click **Login**. Select a patient to log medications out for; then select the drawer you wish to open. Click **Open Drawer**, choose **Put Medication on Tray**, and then click **Close Drawer**.

- Next to the Automated System is a set of drawers identified by patient room number. To access these, click on the drawers themselves or on the **Unit Dosage** icon at the top of the screen. This provides a close-up view of the drawers. Click on the room number of the patient you are working with to open that drawer. Next, click on the medication you would like to prepare for the patient, and a label appears to the right under the patient's name, listing strength, units, and dosage per unit. You can **Open** and **Close** this medication label by clicking the appropriate icon. To exit, click **Close Drawer**; then click **View Medication Room**.

At any time, you can learn about a medication you wish to prepare for a patient by clicking on the **Drug** icon in the bottom left corner of the medication room screen or by clicking the **Drug Guide** book on the counter to the right of the unit dosage drawers. The **Drug Guide** provides information about the medications commonly included in nursing drug handbooks. Nutritional supplements and maintenance intravenous fluid preparations are not included.

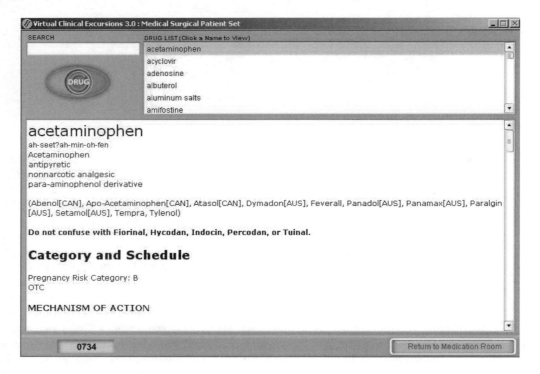

To access the MAR to review the medications ordered for a patient, click on the **MAR** icon located in the tool bar at the top of your screen. You may also click the **Review MAR** icon in the tool bar at the bottom of your screen from inside each medication storage area.

After you have chosen and prepared your medications, return to the patient's room to administer them by clicking on the room number in the bottom tool bar. Once inside the patient's room, click on **Medication Administration** and follow the administration sequence.

■ PRECEPTOR'S EVALUATIONS

When you have finished a session, click on **Leave the Floor** to go to the Floor Menu. At this point, you can click on the icon next to **Look at your Preceptor's Evaluation** to receive a scorecard that provides feedback on the work you completed during patient care.

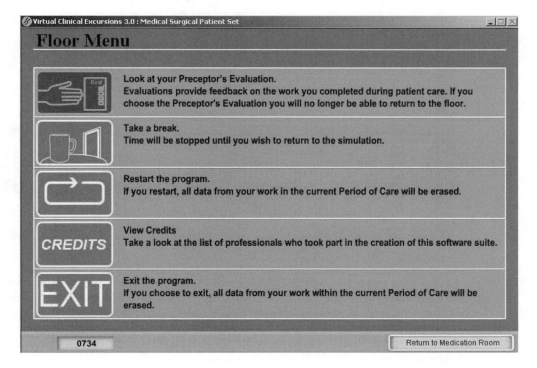

Evaluations are available for each patient you signed in for. Click on any of the **Medication Scorecard** icons to see an example. The scorecard compares the medications you administered to a patient during a period of care with what should have been administered. Table A lists the correct medications. Table B lists any medications that were administered incorrectly.

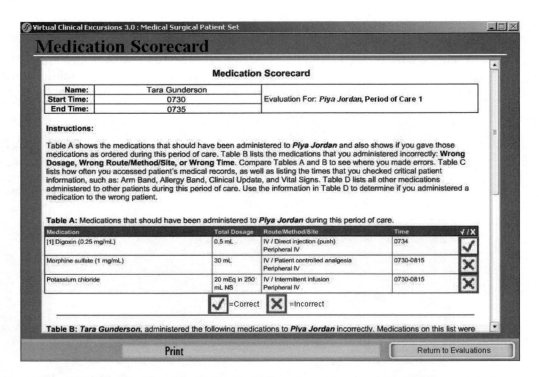

Not every medication listed on the MAR should be given. For example, a patient might have an allergy to a drug that was ordered, or a medication might have been improperly transcribed to the MAR. Predetermined medication "errors" embedded within the program challenge you to exercise critical thinking skills and professional judgment when deciding to administer a medication, just as you would in a real hospital. Use all your available resources, such as the patient's chart and the MAR, to make your decision.

Table C lists the resources that were available to assist you in medication administration, and it documents whether and when you accessed these resources. For example, did you check the patient armband or perform a check of vital signs? If so, when?

You can click **Print** to get a copy of this report if needed. Click **Return to Evaluations** when finished.

■ FLOOR MAP

To get a general sense of your location within the hospital, click on the **Map** icon found in the lower right corner of most of the screens in the *Virtual Clinical Excursions—General Hospital* program. A floor map will appear, showing the layout of the floor you are currently on, as well as a directory of the patients and services on that floor. As you move your cursor over the directory list, the location of each room is highlighted (and vice versa). The floor map can be accessed from the Nurses' Station, Medication Room, and each patient's room.

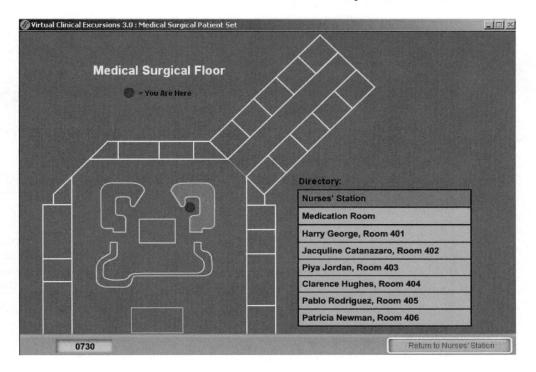

A DETAILED TOUR

If you wish to more thoroughly understand the capabilities of *Virtual Clinical Excursions—General Hospital*, take a detailed tour by completing the following section. During this tour, we will work with a specific patient to introduce you to all the different components and learning opportunities available within the software.

■ WORKING WITH A PATIENT

Sign in and select the Medical-Surgical floor for Period of Care 1 (0730-0815). From the Patient List, select Piya Jordan in Room 403; however, do not go to the Nurses' Station yet.

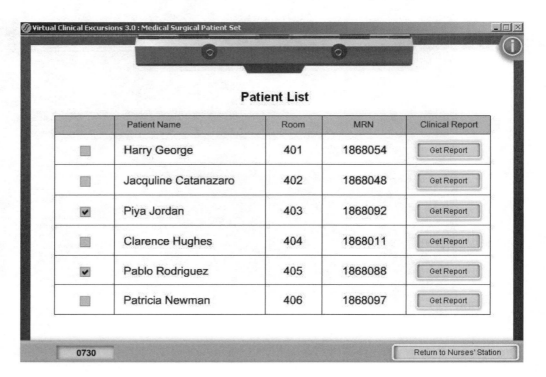

■ REPORT

In hospitals, when one shift ends and another begins, the outgoing nurse who attended a patient will give a verbal and sometimes a written summary of that patient's condition to the incoming nurse who will assume care for the patient. This summary is called a report and is an important source of data to provide an overview of a patient. Your first task is to get clinical report on Piya Jordan. To do this, click **Get Report** in the far right column in this patient's row. From this summary, identify the problems and areas of concern that you will need to address for this patient.

When you have finished reading the report and noting any areas of concern, click on **Return to Patient List** and then on **Go to Nurses' Station**.

■ **CHARTS**

You can access Piya Jordan's chart from the Nurses' Station or from the patient's room (403). We will access it from the Nurses' Station: Click on the chart rack or on the **Chart** icon in the tool bar at the top of your screen. Next, click on the chart labeled **403** to open the medical record for Piya Jordan. Click on the **Emergency Department** tab to view a record of why this patient was admitted.

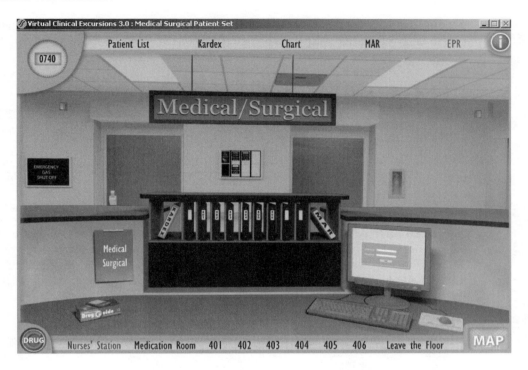

How many days has Piya Jordan been in the hospital?

What tests were done upon her arrival in the Emergency Department and why?

What was her reason for admission?

You should also click on **Surgical Reports** to learn what procedures were performed and when. Finally, review the **Nursing Admission** and **History and Physical** tabs to view information on the health history of this patient. When you are done reviewing the chart, click **Return to Nurses' Station**.

■ MEDICATIONS

Open the Medication Administration Record (MAR) by clicking on the **MAR** icon in the tool bar at the top of your screen. *Remember:* The MAR automatically opens to the first occupied room number on the floor (in this case, Room 401, Harry George). Since you need to access Piya Jordan's MAR, click on tab **403** (her room number). Always make sure you are giving the *Right Drug to the Right Patient!*

Examine the list of medications prescribed for Piya Jordan. Write down the medications that need to be given during this period of care (0730-0815). For each medication, note the dosage, route, and time in the chart below.

Time	Medication	Dosage	Route
0800	Digoxin	0.125 mg	IV

Click on **Return to Nurses' Station**. Next, click on **403** on the bottom tool bar and then verify that you are indeed in Piya Jordan's room. Select **Clinical Alerts** (the icon to the right of Initial Observations) to check for any emerging data that might affect your medication administration priorities. Go to the patient's chart (click on the **Chart** icon; then click on **403**). When the chart opens, select the **Physician's Orders** tab.

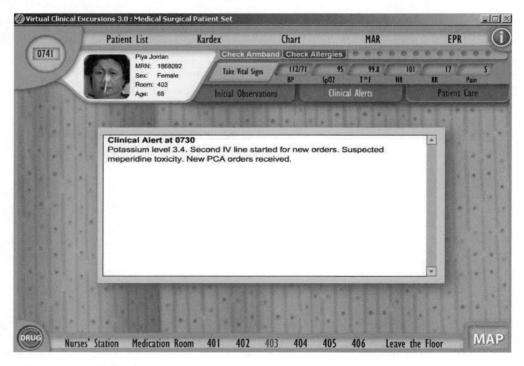

Review the orders. Have any new medications been ordered? Return to the MAR (click **Return to Room 403**; then click **MAR**). Verify that the new medications have been correctly transcribed to the MAR. Mistakes are sometimes made in the transcription process in the hospital setting, and it is sound practice to double-check any new order.

Are there any patient assessments you will need to perform before administering these medications? If so, return to Room 403 and click on **Review of Systems** to complete those before proceeding. (*Hint:* Check apical pulse.)

Now click on the **Medication Room** icon in the tool bar at the bottom of your screen to locate and prepare the medications for Piya Jordan.

In the Medication Room, you must access the medications for Piya Jordan from the specific dispensing system in which each medication is stored. Locate each medication that needs to be given in this time period and click on **Put Medication on Tray** as appropriate. (*Hint:* Look in Unit Dosage drawer first.) When you are finished, click on **Close Drawer** and then on **View Medication Room**. Now click on the medication tray on the counter on the left side of the medication room screen to begin preparing the medications you have selected. (*Note:* Instead of clicking on the tray, you can click **Preparation** at top of screen.)

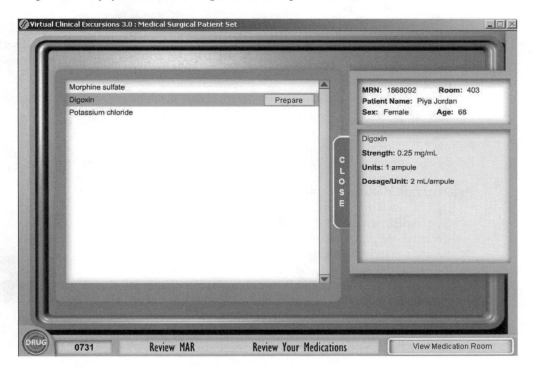

In the preparation area, you should see a list of the medications you put on the tray in the previous steps. Click on the first medication and then click **Prepare**. Follow the onscreen instructions of the Preparation Wizard, providing any data requested. As an example, let's follow the preparation process for digoxin, one of the medications due to be administered to Piya Jordan during this period of care. To begin, click to select **Digoxin**; then click **Prepare**. Now work through the Preparation Wizard sequence as detailed below:

> Amount of medication in the ampule: 2 mL
> Enter the amount of medication you will draw up into a syringe: **0.5** mL
> Click **Next**.
> Select the patient you wish to set aside the medication for:
> Click **Room 403, Piya Jordan**.
> Click **Finish**.
> Click **Return to Medication Room**.

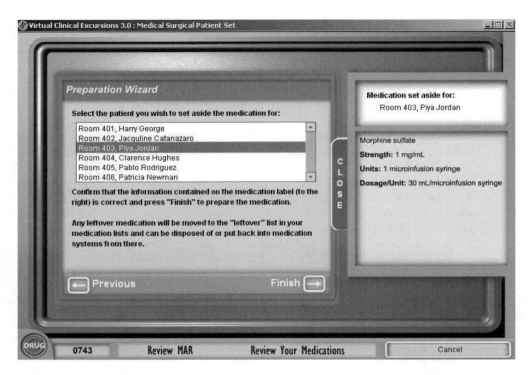

Follow this same basic process for the other medications due to be administered to Piya Jordan during this period of care. (*Hint:* Look in **IV Storage** and **Automated System**.)

PREPARATION WIZARD EXCEPTIONS

- Some medications in *Virtual Clinical Excursions—General Hospital* are preprepared by the pharmacy (e.g., IV antibiotics) and taken to the patient room as a whole. This is common practice in most hospitals.
- Blood products are not administered by students through the *Virtual Clinical Excursions—General Hospital* simulations since blood administration follows specific protocols not covered in this program.
- The *Virtual Clinical Excursions—General Hospital* simulations do not allow for mixing more than one type of medication, such as regular and Lente insulins, in the same syringe. In the clinical setting, when multiple types of insulin are ordered for a patient, the regular insulin is drawn up first, followed by the longer-acting insulin. Insulin is always administered in a special unit-marked syringe.

Now return to Room 403 (click on **403** on bottom tool bar) to administer Piya Jordan's medications.

At any time during the medication administration process, you can perform a further review of systems, take vital signs, check information contained within the chart, or verify patient identity and allergies. Inside Piya Jordan's room, click **Take Vital Signs**. (*Note:* These findings change over time to reflect the temporal changes you would find in a patient similar to Piya Jordan.)

When you have gathered all the data you need, click on **Patient Care** and then select **Medication Administration**. After reviewing your medications, continue the administration process with the digoxin ordered for Piya Jordan. In the list of medications set aside for this patient, click to highlight **Digoxin**. Next, click on the down arrow to the right of **Select** and choose **Administer** from the drop-down menu. This will activate the Administration Wizard. Complete the Wizard sequence as follows:

- Route: **IV**
- Method: **Direct Injection**
- Site: **Peripheral IV**
- Click **Administer to Patient** arrow.
- Would you like to document this administration in the MAR? **Yes**
- Click **Finish** arrow.

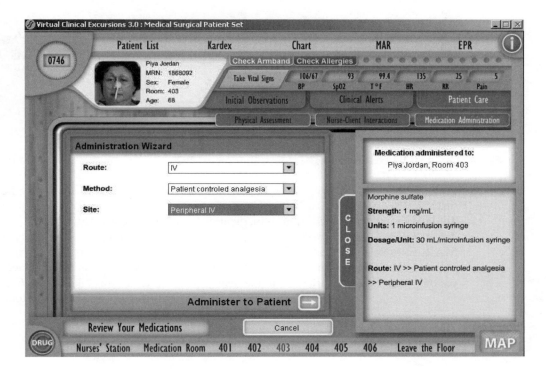

Selections are recorded by a tracking system and evaluated on a Medication Scorecard stored under Preceptor's Evaluations. This scorecard can be viewed, printed, and given to your instructor. To access the Preceptor's Evaluations, click on **Leave the Floor**. When the Floor Menu appears, click on the icon next to **Look at Your Preceptor's Evaluation**. From the list of evaluations, click on **Medication Scorecard** inside the box with Piya Jordan's name.

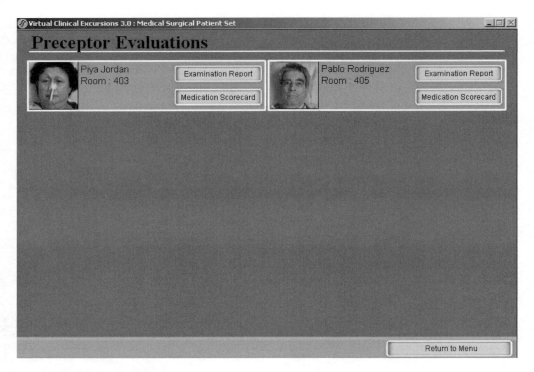

■ MEDICATION SCORECARD

- First, review Table A. Was digoxin given correctly? Did you give the other medications as ordered?
- Table B shows you which (if any) medications you gave incorrectly.
- Table C addresses the resources used for Piya Jordan. Did you access the patient's chart, MAR, EPR, or Kardex as needed to make safe medication administration decisions?
- Did you check the patient's armband to verify her identity? Did you check whether your patient had any known allergies to medications? Were vital signs taken?

■ **VITAL SIGNS**

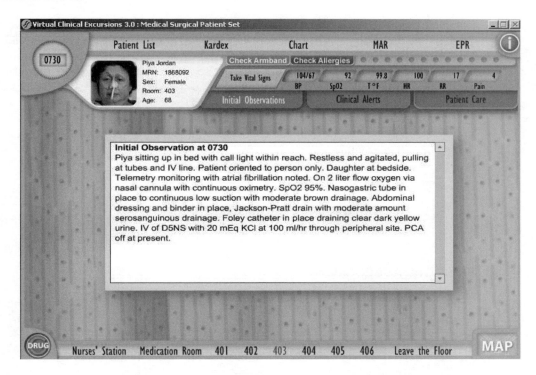

Vital signs, often considered the traditional signs of life, include body temperature, heart rate, respiratory rate, blood pressure, oxygen saturation of the blood, and the patient's experience of pain.

Inside Piya Jordan's room, click **Take Vital Signs**. (*Remember:* You can take vital signs at any time. The data change over time to reflect the temporal changes you would find in a patient similar to Piya Jordan.) Collect vital signs for this patient and record them in the following table. Note the time at which you collected each of these data.

Vital Signs	Findings/Time
Blood pressure	
O$_2$ saturation	
Heart rate	
Respiratory rate	
Temperature	
Pain rating	

After you are done, click on the **EPR** icon located in the tool bar at the top of the screen.

Complete the EPR Login screen as directed in *A Quick Tour* (see page 15 of this workbook). Click on the down arrow next to Patient and choose Piya Jordan's room number **403**. Select **Vital Signs** as the category. Next, record the vital signs data you just collected in the last column. (*Note:* If you need help with this process, see page 16.) Now compare these findings with the data you collected earlier for this patient's vital signs. Use these earlier findings to establish a baseline for each of the vital signs.

a. Are any of the data you collected significantly different from the baseline for a particular vital sign?

Circle One: Yes   No

b. If "Yes," which data are different?

PHYSICAL ASSESSMENT

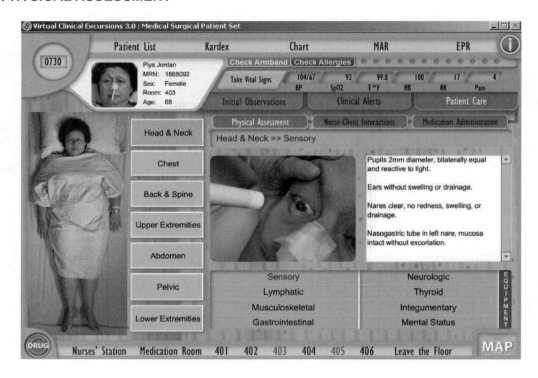

After you have finished examining the EPR for vital signs, click **Exit EPR** to return to Room 403. Click **Patient Care** and then **Physical Assessment**. Think about what information you received in report, as well as what you may have learned about this patient from the chart. What area(s) of examination should you pay most attention to at this time? Is there any equipment you should be monitoring? Conduct a physical assessment of the body areas and systems that you consider priorities for Piya Jordan. For example, select **Head & Neck**; then click on and assess **Sensory** and **Lymphatic**. Complete any other assessment(s) you think are necessary at this time. In the following table, record the data you collected during this examination.

Area of Examination	Findings
Head & Neck Sensory	
Head & Neck Lymphatic	

After you have finished collecting these data, return to the EPR. Compare the data that were already in the record with those you just collected.

    a.   Are any of the data you collected significantly different from the baselines for this patient?

           Circle One: Yes   No

    b.   If "Yes," which data are different?

■ **NURSE-CLIENT INTERACTIONS**

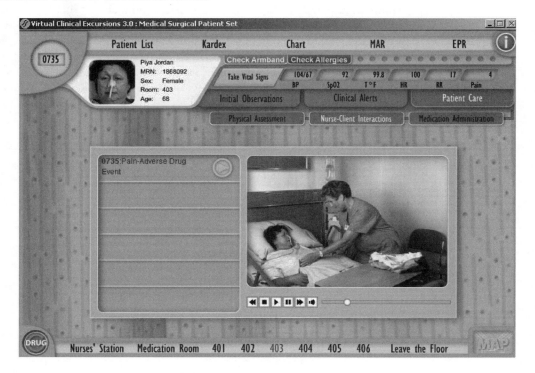

Click on **Patient Care** from inside Piya Jordan's room (403). Now click on **Nurse-Client Interactions** to access a short video titled **Pain—Adverse Drug Event**, which is available for viewing at 0735 (based on the virtual clock in the upper left corner of your screen). To begin the video, click on the arrow next to its title. You will observe a nurse communicating with Piya Jordan and her daughter. There are many variations of nursing practice, some exemplifying "best" practice and some not. Note whether the nurse in this interaction displays professional behavior and compassionate care. Are her words congruent with what is going on with the patient? Does this interaction "feel right" to you? If not, how would you handle this situation differently? Explain.

Note: If the video you wish to view is not listed, this means you have not yet reached the correct virtual time to view that video. Check the virtual clock; you may return to access the video once its designated time has occurred—as long as you do so within the corresponding period of care.

At least one Nurse-Client Interactions video is available during each period of care. Viewing these videos can help you learn more about what is occurring with a patient at a certain time and also prompt you to discriminate between nurse communications that are ideal and those that need improvement. Compassionate care and the ability to communicate clearly are essential components of delivering quality nursing care, and it is during your clinical time that you will begin to refine these skills.

■ COLLECTING AND EVALUATING DATA

Each of the activities you perform in the Patient Care environment generates a great deal of assessment data. Remember that after you collect data, you can record your findings in the EPR. You can also review the EPR, patient's chart, videos, and MAR at any time. You will get plenty of practice collecting and then evaluating data in context of the patient's course.

Now, here's an important question for you:

> Did the previous sequence of exercises provide the most efficient way to assess Piya Jordan?

For example, you went to the patient's room to get vital signs, then back to the EPR to enter data and compare your findings with extant data. Next, you went back to the patient's room to do a physical examination, then again back to the EPR to enter and review data. If this back-and-forth process of data collection and recording seemed inefficient, remember the following:

- Plan all of your nursing activities to maximize efficiency while at the same time optimizing quality of patient care. (Think about what data you might need to perform certain tasks. For example, do you need to check a heart rate before administering a cardiac medication or check an IV site before starting an infusion?)

- You collect a tremendous amount of data when you work with a patient. Very few people can accurately remember all these data for more than a few minutes. Develop efficient assessment skills, and record data as soon as possible after collecting them.

- Assessment data are only the starting point for the nursing process.

Make a clear distinction between these first exercises and how you actually provide nursing care. These initial exercises were designed to involve you actively in the use of different software components. This workbook focuses on sensible practices for implementing the nursing process in ways that ensure the highest quality care of patients.

Most important, remember that a human being changes through time, and that these changes include both the physical and psychosocial facets of a person as a living organism. Think about this for a moment. Some patients may change physically in a very short time (a patient with emerging myocardial infarction) or more slowly (a patient with a chronic illness). Patients' overall physical and psychosocial conditions may improve or deteriorate. They may have effective coping skills and familial support, or they may feel alone and full of despair. In fact, each individual is a complex mix of physical and psychosocial elements, and at least some of these elements usually change through time.

Thus it is crucial *not* to think of the nursing process as a simple one-time, five-step procedure:

- Assessment
- Nursing Diagnosis
- Planning
- Implementation
- Evaluation

Rather, the nursing process should be utilized as a creative and systematic approach to delivering nursing care. Furthermore, because all living organisms are constantly changing, we must apply the nursing process over and over. Each time we follow the nursing process for an individual patient, we refine our understanding of that patient's physical and psychosocial conditions based on collection and analysis of many different types of data. *Virtual Clinical Excursions—General Hospital* will help you develop both the creativity and the systematic approach needed to become a nurse who is equipped to deliver the highest quality care to all patients.

REDUCING MEDICATION ERRORS

Earlier in this detailed tour, you learned the basic steps of medication preparation and administration. The following simulations will allow you to practice those skills further—with an increased emphasis on reducing medication errors by using the Medication Scorecard to evaluate your work.

Sign in to work at Pacific View Regional Hospital for Period of Care 1. (*Note:* If you are already working with another patient or during another period of care, click on **Leave the Floor** and then **Restart the Program**; then sign in.)

From the Patient List, select Clarence Hughes. Then click on **Go To Nurses' Station**. Complete the following steps to prepare and administer medications to Clarence Hughes.

- Click on **Medication Room**.
- Click on **MAR** to determine prn medications that have been ordered for Clarence Hughes to address his constipation and pain. (*Note:* You may click on **Review MAR** at any time to verify correct medication order. Remember to look at the patient name on the MAR to make sure you have the correct patient's record—you must click on the correct room number within the MAR.) Click on **Return to Medication Room** after reviewing the correct MAR.
- Click on **Unit Dosage** (or on the Unit Dosage cabinet); from the close-up view, click on drawer **404**.
- Select the medications you would like to administer. After each selection, click **Put Medication on Tray**. When you are finished selecting medications, click **Close Drawer**.
- Click on **View Medication Room**.
- Click on **Automated System** (or on the Automated System unit itself). Click **Login**.
- On the next screen, specify the correct patient and drawer location.
- Select the medication you would like to administer and click on **Put Medication on Tray**. Repeat this process if you wish to administer other medications from the Automated System.
- When you are finished, click **Close Drawer**. At the bottom right corner of the next screen, click on **View Medication Room**.
- From the Medication Room, click on **Preparation** (or on the preparation tray).
- From the list of medications on your tray, choose the correct medication to administer.
- Click **Next**, specify the correct patient to administer this medication to, and click **Finish**.
- Repeat the previous two steps until all medications that you want to administer are prepared.
- You can click on **Review Your Medications** and then on **Return to Medication Room** when ready. Once you are back in the Medication Room, go directly to Clarence Hughes' room by clicking on **404** at bottom of screen.
- Inside the patient's room, administer the medication, utilizing the five rights of medication administration. After you have collected the appropriate assessment data and are ready for administration, click **Patient Care** and then **Medication Administration**. Verify that the correct patient and medication(s) appear in the left-hand window. Then click the down arrow next to Select. From the drop-down menu, select **Administer** and complete the Administration Wizard by providing any information requested. When the Wizard stops asking for information, click **Administer to Patient**. Specify **Yes** when asked whether this administration should be recorded in the MAR. Finally, click **Finish**.

■ SELF-EVALUATION

Now let's see how you did during your earlier medication administration!

- Click on **Leave the Floor** at the bottom of your screen. From the Floor Menu, select **Look at Your Preceptor's Evaluation**. Then click on **Medication Scorecard**.

These resources will help you find out more about each patient's medications and possible sources of medication errors.

1. Start by examining Table A. These are the medications you should have given to Clarence Hughes during this period of care. If each of the medications in Table A has a ✓ by it, then you made no errors. Congratulations!

If there are some medications that have an X by them, then you made one or more medication errors.

Compare Tables A and B to determine which of the following types of errors you made: Wrong Dose, Wrong Route/Method/Site, or Wrong Time. Follow these steps:
   a. Find medications in Table A that were given incorrectly.
   b. Now see if those same medications are in Table B, which shows what you actually administered to Clarence Hughes.
   c. Comparing Tables A and B, match the Strength, Dose, Route/Method/Site, and Time for each medication you administered incorrectly.
   d. Then, using the form below, list the medications given incorrectly and mark the errors you made for each medication.

Medication	Strength	Dosage	Route	Method	Site	Time
	❑	❑	❑	❑	❑	❑
	❑	❑	❑	❑	❑	❑
	❑	❑	❑	❑	❑	❑
	❑	❑	❑	❑	❑	❑

2. To help you reduce future medication errors, consider the following list of possible reasons for errors.

- Did not check drug against MAR for correct patient, correct date, correct time, correct drug, and correct dose.
- Did not check drug dose against MAR three times.
- Did not open the unit dose package in the patient's room.
- Did not correctly identify the patient using two identifiers.
- Did not administer the drug on time.
- Did not verify patient allergies.
- Did not check the patient's current condition or vital sign parameters.
- Did not consider why the patient would be receiving this drug.
- Did not question why the drug was in the patient's drawer.
- Did not check the physician's order and/or check with the pharmacist when there was a question about the drug or dose.
- Did not verify that no adverse effects had occurred from a previous dose.

Based on these possibilities, determine how you made each error and record the reason into the form below:

Medication	Reason for Error

3. Look again at Table B. Are there medications listed that are not in Table A? If so, you gave a medication to Clarence Hughes that he should not have received. Complete the following exercises to help you understand how such an error might have been made.

   a. Perhaps you gave a medication that was on Clarence Hughes' MAR for this period of care, without recognizing that a change had occurred in the patient's condition that should have caused you to reconsider. Review patient records as necessary and complete the following form:

Medication	Possible Reasons Not to Give This Medication

   b. Another possibility is that you gave Clarence Hughes a medication that should have been given at a different time. Check his MAR and complete the form below to determine whether you made a Wrong Time error:

Medication	Given to Clarence Hughes at What Time	Should Have Been Given at What Time

c. Maybe you gave another patient's medication to Clarence Hughes. In this case, you made a Wrong Patient error. Check the MARs of other patients and use the form below to determine whether you made this type of error:

Medication	Given to Clarence Hughes	Should Have Been Given to

4. The Medication Scorecard provides some other interesting sources of information. For example, if there is a medication selected for Clarence Hughes but it was not given to him, there will be an X by that medication in Table A, but it will not appear in Table B. In that case, you might have given this medication to some other patient, which is another type of Wrong Patient error. To investigate further, look at Table D, which lists the medications you gave to other patients. See whether you can find any medications for Clarence Hughes that were given to another patient by mistake. Before making any decisions, be sure to cross-check the other patients' MAR because they may have had the same medication ordered. Use the following form to record your findings:

Medication	Should Have Been Given to Clarence Hughes	Given by Mistake to

5. Now take some time to review the exercises you just completed. Use the form below to create an overall analysis of what you have learned. Once again, record each of the medication errors you made, including the type of each error. Then, for each error you made, indicate specifically what you would do differently to prevent this type of error from occurring again.

Medication	Type of Error	Error Prevention Tactic

Submit this form to your instructor if required as a graded assignment, or simply use these exercises to improve your understanding of medication errors and how to reduce them.

Name: _____   Date: _____

The following icons are used throughout the workbook to help you quickly identify particular activities and assignments:

 Indicates a reading assignment—tells you which textbook chapter(s) you should read before starting each lesson

 Indicates a writing activity

 Marks the beginning of an interactive CD-ROM activity—signals you to open or return to your *Virtual Clinical Excursions—General Hospital* CD-ROM

 Indicates additional CD-ROM instructions

 Indicates questions and activities that require you to consult your textbook

 Indicates the approximate time required to complete an exercise

 Indicates a link to another exercise or lesson with this same patient

LESSON **1** _____

Critical Thinking and Nursing Judgment

_____

⁓ **Reading Assignment:**   Critical Thinking and Nursing Judgment (Chapter 6)
Nursing Process (Chapter 7)

Patient: Harry George, Medical-Surgical Floor, Room 401

Objectives:

- Identify how to apply critical thinking to the assessment of a patient.
- Discuss ways to use reflection when preparing for patient care.
- Identify examples of critical thinking attitudes applied in the assessment of patients in the case studies.
- Describe how intellectual standards apply in patient assessment.
- Identify examples of professional standards to use in patient care.
- Apply a critical thinking model to the assessment of patients in the case studies.

Each patient experience poses new opportunities and problems involving patient care. In each clinical situation, you have the responsibility to think critically and make sound clinical decisions. During any patient encounter, you must use the skills of critical thinking: applying the nursing process, recalling past experiences that can help in the care of your current patient, reflecting on the knowledge that applies to a patient's health situation, applying intellectual standards and critical thinking attitudes, and exercising professional standards of practice.

The challenge of clinical decision making is rewarding and fulfilling. Each patient presents a unique clinical picture that requires you to observe and examine the patient closely, search for patterns of patient problems, consider scientific principles relating to patient problems, recognize the problems and develop a plan of care, and then act on the plan and evaluate results. Ultimately, the use of critical thinking in patient care enables you to find the solutions that best support and help your patient towards an improved level of health.

Exercise 1

 CD-ROM Activity

 45 minutes

In this exercise you will visit Harry George, a 42-year-old Caucasian male who was admitted to the hospital with symptoms of infection and swelling of the foot. He has a history of abusing alcohol. He has been diagnosed with cellulitis and osteomyelitis of the foot. You may have worked with Harry George previously if you already completed Lesson 16 or 18.

- Sign in to work at Pacific View Regional Hospital on the Medical-Surgical Floor for Period of Care 1. (*Note:* If you are already in the virtual hospital from a previous exercise, click on **Leave the Floor** and then **Restart the Program** to get to the sign-in window.)
- From the Patient List, select Harry George (Room 401).
- Click on **Get Report**.
- Click on **Go to Nurses' Station**.
- Click on **Chart**.
- Select the chart for Room **401**.
- Click on and review the **Nursing Admission**.

1. Fill in the following form by completing each category as you review the Nursing Admission history for Harry George.

Reason for Admission/Chief Complaint

Nutrition/Metabolic

Skin

Activity/Rest

Self-Perception

Pain

• Review the nurse's admission description of the patient's left leg wound.
  • Next, click on **Consultations** and review the note from the wound care team.

2. Intellectual standards of critical thinking are commonly applied when assessing a patient. Compare the Nursing Admission description of Harry George's left foot in the progress note with the description in the wound care consultation.

   a. Which note was more complete? Explain.

   b. The wound care team reported the wound at 3 cm, whereas the nurse's note reported 2 cm. How would you validate the assessment finding?

   c. In what way was the wound care team's consultation note more precise?

 3. What objective professional standard was used in the assessment of Harry George's pain? (*Study Tip:* Review pages 845-850 in your textbook.)

4. After collecting assessment data and validating for accuracy, you begin to interpret the clinical information by organizing it into meaningful:
   a. inferences.
   b. problems.
   c. clusters.
   d. nursing diagnoses.

 • Click on **Return to Nurses' Station**.
  • Click on the computer screen.
  • Click on **EPR** and **Login**.
  • Specify **401** as the patient's room and **Vital Signs** as the category.
  • Review the data from Monday at 1835 up to Wednesday 0700.
  • Now change the category to **Nutrition** and review these data for the same time frame.

5. Certain cues will usually alert you to patterns that suggest a nursing diagnosis. After reviewing data from the nursing history and EPR, match the defining characteristics on the left with data clusters from Harry George's admission history on the right.

Defining Characteristics	Admission Data
_____ Verbal report	a. Change in sleep cycle
_____ Sore inflamed buccal cavity	b. Groans
_____ Lack of interest in food	c. Eats one meal a day
_____ Expressive behavior	d. "My foot is killing me"
_____ Sleep disturbance	e. Gums dark pink, swollen
_____ Reported food intake less than RDA	f. "Haven't felt like eating for last week"

6. As a nurse puts together cues, patterns emerge in the form of nursing diagnoses. Sometimes cues for more than one nursing diagnosis overlap. In the case of Harry George, his sleep disturbance might indicate the effects of the diagnosis Pain or it could be a defining characteristic for the diagnosis Disturbed Sleep Pattern. As a critical thinker, what would you do to clarify and be sure data were interpreted correctly?

7. As the nurse, you review the Activity/Rest portion of the Nursing Admission history. The sleep pattern is documented as being "irregular, never more than 2 hours." Your decision to question the patient further about the sleep habits he follows—time he normally goes to bed, activities prior to going to sleep, and number of awakenings during night—is an example of what critical thinking attitude?
   a. Humility
   b. Thinking independently
   c. Risk taking
   d. Perseverance

 • Click on **Return to Nurses' Station**.
   • Click on **Chart**.
   • Select the chart for Room **401**.
   • Click on and read the **History and Physical**.
   • Review the physician's plan.

8. Critical thinking involves the application of knowledge in order to fully analyze and understand a patient's problems. Given the physician's medical plan, list four areas of knowledge that would help you in supporting the plan of care.

• Click on **Return to Nurses' Station**.
  • Select **401** at the bottom of the screen to visit the patient's room.
  • Click on **Patient Care**.
  • Select **Lower Extremities** and review the assessment findings.

Fill in the blanks with the critical thinking concepts that best describe the following situations.

  9. After reviewing the condition of Harry George's wound, the conclusion as to whether the

     wound is healing is an example of _____ _____.

 10. When you see a change in a wound from reddened margins to clear and less inflamed, you

     make an _____ from this evidence in order to conclude the wound is healing.

 11. After applying saline to Harry George's wound over 2 days, your evaluation of the use of

     saline over time is an example of _____ _____.

 12. If you, as the nurse, questioned the wound care team's recommendations for a dressing for
     Harry George, you would be demonstrating the critical thinking attitude of

     _____ _____.

Exercise 2

 CD-ROM Activity

  45 minutes

In this exercise you will visit Harry George, a 42-year-old Caucasian male who was admitted to the hospital with symptoms of infection and swelling of the foot. He has a history of abusing alcohol. He has been diagnosed with cellulitis and osteomyelitis of the foot. You may have worked with Harry George previously if you already completed Exercise 1 or Lesson 16 or 18.

  • Sign in to work at Pacific View Regional Hospital on the Medical-Surgical Floor for Period
    of Care 4. (*Note:* If you are already in the virtual hospital from a previous exercise, click on
    Leave the Floor and then **Restart the Program** to get to the sign-in window.)
  • From the Patient List, select Harry George (Room 401).
  • Click on **Get Report**.
  • Click on **Go to Nurses' Station**.
  • Click on **Chart**.
  • Select the chart for Room **401**.
  • Click on and review the **Nursing Admission**.
  • Click on and review the **Nurse's Notes** from 1200 Wednesday through 1900 Wednesday.
  • Next, click on **Consultations** and read the note from the Psychiatric Consult.
  • Finally, review the **Physician's Notes**.

1. Harry George has experienced the loss of his family and admits that his drinking problem has become serious. Critical thinking applied to assessment enables a nurse to develop a relevant plan of care. Complete the following critical thinking diagram for assessment of Harry George's situation by writing the letter of each critical thinking factor under its proper category.

Knowledge

1. _____

2. _____

3. _____

Experience   **Standards**

4. _____   **ASSESSMENT**   6. _____
                   SELF-CONCEPT
5. _____   7. _____

                   Attitudes

8. _____

9. _____

Critical Thinking Factors

a. Review the principles of self-concept.
b. Ask Harry George to discuss his relationship with his parents and its effects on his ability to cope with the loss of his immediate family.
c. Apply principles of therapeutic communication in building a trusting relationship with Harry George.
d. Apply what you have learned from caring for patients with depression in the past to Harry George's case.
e. During your interview with Harry George, apply the criteria of phases of grief in determining the extent of his loss and take time to be thorough in your assessment.
f. When assessing Harry George's perception of self-concept, pay attention to his behavior and the content of his conversation.
g. Reflect on those situations when you have had to deal with agitated and restless patients.
h. Consider what you know about symptoms and etiology of alcohol withdrawal.
i. Stay focused on the best interests of Harry George; keep him as comfortable as possible, managing his symptoms while attempting to assess his needs.

2. When gathering a nursing health history, there are five health dimensions for gathering data. List those dimensions.

3. When analyzing the data about Harry George's self-concept and family relationships, critical thinking ensures a complete data base. Match the critical thinking attitude on the left with the assessment approach on the right.

Critical Thinking Attitude	**Assessment Approach**
_____ Significant	a. During each encounter, observe the patient's facial expression and bodily movement.
_____ Consistent	b. Inquire "Mr. George, what does the loss of your family mean to you?"
_____ Accurate	c. Ask, "Mr. George, clarify for me, what exactly happened prior to your wife deciding to leave you?"

LESSON 2

Applying the Nursing Process

👓 **Reading Assignment:** Nursing Process (Chapter 7)

Patient: Patricia Newman, Medical-Surgical Floor, Room 406

Objectives:

- Assess the health care needs of patients in the case studies.
- Analyze data clusters from data gathered in nursing assessment.
- Develop nursing diagnoses from data presented in the case studies.
- Identify relationship of nursing diagnoses in a concept map.
- Identify priorities of nursing care for a case study patient.
- Develop goal and outcome statements.
- Discuss factors to consider in choosing nursing interventions.
- Identify types of nursing interventions.
- Evaluate status of patients in the case studies.

Each time you care for a patient, you apply the nursing process. The process begins with your assessment of a patient's health status. Analysis and interpretation of assessment data lead to the formation of nursing diagnoses and collaborative problems. After identifying relevant nursing diagnoses, you develop a plan of care. The plan directs how you implement the patient's care, using direct and indirect interventions. After administering interventions, you evaluate the patient's response and progress towards an improved level of health. The nursing process provides a framework to apply critical thinking skills in making competent decisions about the care of all patients.

Exercise 1

 CD-ROM Activity

 30 minutes

 In this exercise you will visit Patricia Newman, a 61-year-old Caucasian female who has a history of emphysema, osteoporosis, and hypertension. She has been admitted to the hospital in moderate respiratory distress. You may have worked with Patricia Newman previously if you already completed Lesson 2, 3, 5, 9, or 10.

- Sign in to work at Pacific View Regional Hospital on the Medical-Surgical Floor for Period of Care 1. (*Note:* If you are already in the virtual hospital from a previous exercise, click on **Leave the Floor** and then **Restart the Program** to get to the sign-in window.)
- From the Patient List, select Patricia Newman (Room 406).
- Click on **Get Report**.
- Click on **Go to Nurses' Station**.
- Click on **Chart**.
- Select the chart for Room **406**.

1. Nursing assessment involves the careful review, analysis, and interpretation of data about a patient's health status. Complete the following assessment flow sheet, based on your review of data for Patricia Newman in the following chart files:

   - Nursing Admission
   - History and Physical

1. Vital signs and blood gases from 0700 clinical report	BP HR RR Temp SpO$_2$ pH PaO$_2$ CO$_3$ CO$_2$
2. History of present illness	
3. Health promotion	Description of health: Usual BP: Flu shot: TB test: Routine self-exam:

4. Nutrition	Appetite: _____ Meals/day: _____
	Fluid intake daily: _____
	Oral cavity: _____
	Other problems:
5. Respiratory	Cough:
	Lung sounds:
	Other symptoms:
6. Cardiovascular	Heart sounds:
	Abnormal findings:
7. Activity/Rest	Energy level:
	Other problems:

2. The patient's statement describing her health as "not very good" is an example of:
   a. objective data.
   b. back channeling.
   c. defining characteristic.
   d. subjective data.

3. The measurement of objective data is based on accepted standards. For each of the following findings from Patricia Newman's assessment, identify the standard used in measurement.

Lung sounds

Temperature

Oral cavity

4. After reviewing the findings for Patricia Newman's cardiovascular and respiratory status, what other sources of similar data might you use? List two.

 • Click on **Return to Nurses' Station**.
• Select Room **406** at the bottom of the screen.
• Review the **Initial Observations**.
• Click on **Patient Care**.
• Click on and review the examination findings for the **Chest** and then for the **Back & Spine**.

5. Data you gather from a physical assessment help to confirm and broaden the data you have about potential problem areas. After reviewing assessment data on Patricia Newman, what problems are you beginning to identify? List three.

6. Data clusters are sets of signs or symptoms that are grouped together logically. Match the sign or symptom with the appropriate data cluster "categories" listed.

Signs and Symptoms	**Data Cluster**
_____ Reduced energy level	a. Respiratory/Oxygenation
_____ Dyspnea on exertion	b. Reduced Energy Level
_____ Productive cough	
_____ Oxygen saturation 92%	
_____ Feels "too tired to do much"	
_____ Requires frequent rest periods	
_____ Respirations labored	
_____ PaO$_2$ below normal	

7. As you identify clusters of data, you reason to recognize patterns or trends. Data often contain defining characteristics, or criteria, for nursing diagnoses. Listed below are three nursing diagnoses with defining characteristics. Place an X next to all diagnoses that apply to Patricia Newman.

_____ a. Ineffective Airway Clearance: diminished breath sounds, dyspnea, adventitious breath sounds, cough ineffective, sputum production, changes in respiratory rate

_____ b. Impaired Gas Exchange: tachycardia, hypoxia, abnormal arterial blood gases, abnormal rate and depth of breathing, hypoxemia

_____ c. Ineffective Breathing Pattern: pursed-lip breathing, dyspnea, use of accessory muscles to breathe, respiratory rate higher than 24 per minute, altered chest excursion

8. The related factors contributing to Patricia Newman's nursing diagnoses must be accurate for what reason?

9. Which of the following diagnostic statements apply to Patricia Newman? (Place an X next to all that apply.)

_____ a. Impaired Gas Exchange related to abnormal blood gas levels

_____ b. Activity Intolerance related to general weakness

_____ c. Imbalanced Nutrition: Less Than Body Requirements related to patient's need for high-protein diet

_____ d. Impaired Gas Exchange related to alveolar capillary changes

_____ e. Activity Intolerance related to insufficient exercise

_____ f. Imbalanced Nutrition: Less Than Body Requirements related to reduced intake of nutrients

10. Given Patricia Newman's numerous physical problems, develop a concept map by drawing arrows with dotted lines to show association between nursing diagnoses. (*Study Tip:* Review writing concept maps on pages 121-122 in your textbook.)

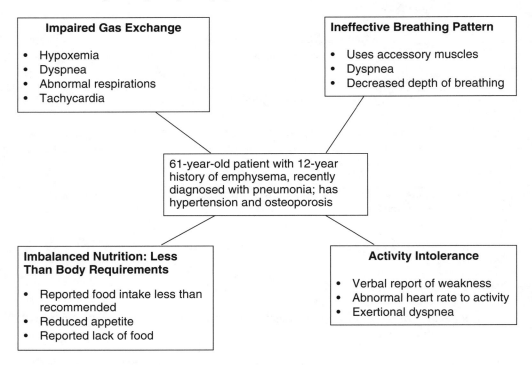

Impaired Gas Exchange

- Hypoxemia
- Dyspnea
- Abnormal respirations
- Tachycardia

Ineffective Breathing Pattern

- Uses accessory muscles
- Dyspnea
- Decreased depth of breathing

61-year-old patient with 12-year history of emphysema, recently diagnosed with pneumonia; has hypertension and osteoporosis

Imbalanced Nutrition: Less Than Body Requirements

- Reported food intake less than recommended
- Reduced appetite
- Reported lack of food

Activity Intolerance

- Verbal report of weakness
- Abnormal heart rate to activity
- Exertional dyspnea

Exercise 2

 CD-ROM Activity

 45 minutes

 In this exercise you will visit Patricia Newman, a 61-year-old Caucasian female who has a history of emphysema, osteoporosis, and hypertension. She has been admitted to the hospital in moderate respiratory distress. You may have worked with Patricia Newman previously if you already completed Exercise 1 of this lesson or if you completed Lesson 3, 9, or 10.

- Sign in to work at Pacific View Regional Hospital on the Medical-Surgical Floor for Period of Care 2. (*Note:* If you are already in the virtual hospital from a previous exercise, click on **Leave the Floor** and then **Restart the Program** to get to the sign-in window.)
- From the Patient List, select Patricia Newman (Room 406).
- Click on **Get Report**.
- Click on **Go to Nurses' Station**.
- Click on **406** to go to the patient's room.
- Review the **Initial Observations.**

1. As you review both the clinical report for 0730 to 1115 and the initial observation in the patient's room, you notice conflicting data. What would be your first action as you begin care for Patricia Newman?
   a. Discuss with her the plan of care for the day
   b. Validate her pulmonary status by conducting a physical examination
   c. Begin instruction on breathing exercises
   d. Call the physician to review data from report

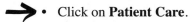 • Click on **Patient Care**.

- Review the list of available assessment categories (yellow buttons), as well as the subcategories of each area (green buttons).

2. Because you want to validate Patricia Newman's pulmonary status, you will conduct a focused assessment. Which assessment categories should you include when examining Patricia Newman? (Place an X next to all that apply.)

Head & Neck

_____ Sensory

_____ Lymphatic

_____ Musculoskeletal

_____ Neurologic

_____ Mental Status

Chest

_____ Integumentary

_____ Cardiovascular

_____ Respiratory

_____ Musculoskeletal

Back & Spine

_____ Integumentary

_____ Musculoskeletal

_____ Respiratory

Abdomen

_____ Musculoskeletal

_____ Gastrointestinal

• Now complete your assessment of the patient based on your answer to question 2.

3. Earlier in Exercise 1, we identified the following nursing diagnoses for Patricia Newman: Impaired Gas Exchange, Ineffective Breathing Pattern, Activity Intolerance, and Imbalanced Nutrition: Less Than Body Requirements. Which of these diagnoses would be validated by your assessment in question 2?

• Click on **Nurse-Client Interactions**.

• Select and view the video titled **1100: Care Coordination**. (*Note:* If this video is not available, check the virtual clock to see whether enough time has elapsed. The video cannot be viewed before its specified time.)

• Click on **Return to the Nurses' Station**.

• Click on **Chart**.

• Select the chart for Room **406**.

• Review the **Physician's Notes**.

4. During the interaction the nurse collected valuable information from Patricia Newman, particularly since the physician has planned a number of consults. Listed below are two possible nursing diagnoses with defining characteristics that might apply to Patricia Newman. Place an X next to the one that you believe might be most appropriate for this patient.

_____ a. Deficient Knowledge regarding appropriate diet (defining characteristics: verbalizes problem, inaccurate follow-through of instruction, inaccurate performance of test, inappropriate behavior)

_____ b. Readiness for Enhanced Knowledge (defining characteristics: expresses an interest in learning, explains knowledge of topic, behaviors congruent with expressed knowledge, describes previous experience pertaining to topic)

5. Provide a rationale for the nursing diagnosis you chose in question 4.

➡ • While still in the chart, review the **History and Physical**.

6. Based on the two nursing diagnoses listed below, write a goal and two expected outcomes for each.

a. Impaired Gas Exchange

   Goal   Expected Outcomes

b. Readiness for Enhanced Knowledge

   Goal   Expected Outcomes

7. It is important to write goals and outcomes clearly. Explain what is inaccurate about each of the following outcome statements.

   a. Respirations will be unlabored with a nonproductive cough

   b. Patient's lung sounds will improve within 24 hours

   c. Patient will feel less tired by discharge

   d. Patient will become afebrile within 24 hours

During the Nurse-Client Interactions, the nurse suggests that social work might be able to assist with resources for smoking cessation and being able to obtain healthy meals for Patricia Newman. Fill in the blanks in the statements below that describe consultation:

8. Consultation is based on the _____ _____ approach.

9. Consultation increases a nurse's _____ about a problem.

10. After a dietitian assesses Patricia Newman's knowledge of food sources and her ability to

    acquire food and prepare meals, the dietitian can more _____ identify the nutritional problem.

11. When making a consultation, it is important for the nurse not to _____ the consultant.

➡ • While still in the chart, review the **Physician's Orders**.

12. In developing a plan of care for Patricia Newman's diagnosis of Impaired Gas Exchange, the nurse selects a series of interventions. Match each intervention with its type. (*Study Tip:* To understand the rationale for the interventions, review textbook Chapter 28.)

Interventions	Type
_____ Administer oxygen at 2 L per nasal cannula	a. Nurse-initiated
	b. Physician-initiated
_____ Instruct patient on how to perform pursed-lip breathing	c. Collaborative
_____ Position patient with head of bed elevated to 45 degrees	
_____ Administer bronchodilator by a metered-dose inhaler	
_____ Have the patient perform cascade coughing every 1 hour	
_____ Encourage oral fluids of 3 L daily	

13. A nurse caring for Patricia Newman performs the following activities. Which of the activities are examples of indirect care measures? (Place an X next to all that apply.)

_____ a. Adjusts the oxygen flow meter to ensure that it runs correctly and checks condition of the tubing

_____ b. Coaches the patient on the technique for performing a cascade cough

_____ c. Documents the character of Patricia Newman's cough and ability to expectorate mucus

_____ d. Consults with the respiratory therapist about the patient's use of a metered-dose inhaler

_____ e. Administers intravenous fluid infusion

14. For each of the expected outcomes listed below, write an evaluation measure.

a. Patient's lungs will clear without crackles within 48 hours

b. Patient's fluid intake will be 3 L every 24 hours

c. Patient will perform pursed-lip breathing correctly within 24 hours

d. Patient will experience less dyspnea while ambulating within 2 days

Exercise 3

 CD-ROM Activity

 30 minutes

 In this exercise you will visit Patricia Newman, a 61-year-old Caucasian female who has a history of emphysema, osteoporosis, and hypertension. She has been admitted to the hospital in moderate respiratory distress. You may have worked with Patricia Newman previously if you already completed Exercise 1 or 2 or Lesson 3 or 9.

- Sign in to work at Pacific View Regional Hospital on the Medical-Surgical Floor for Period of Care 2. (*Note:* If you are already in the virtual hospital from a previous exercise, click on **Leave the Floor** and then **Restart the Program** to get to the sign-in window.)
- From the Patient List, select Patricia Newman (Room 406).
- Click on **Get Report**.

1. As you review the two clinical reports, complete the table below and evaluate the patient's clinical trend as either I (improving), S (remaining stable), or W (worsening).

Findings	0731-1115	1201-1500	Clinical Trend
SpO$_2$			
Blood pressure			
IV site			
Respiratory character			
Lung sounds			

2. Identify the evaluation measure used for each of Patricia Newman's physical findings.

Finding	Evaluation Measure
Lungs less coarse	
IV site without redness	
SpO$_2$	
Respirations shallow	

3. If you already completed Exercise 1 of this lesson, you will remember that Patricia Newman had two nursing diagnoses for her respiratory problems: Impaired Gas Exchange and Ineffective Breathing Pattern. Listed below are two outcomes that apply to each of the diagnoses.

Diagnosis	Outcomes
Impaired Gas Exchange	Patient will have a reduction in heart rate
	Patient will have an improved SpO$_2$
Ineffective Breathing Pattern	Patient will report less breathlessness
	Respirations will be less labored

Based on the clinical report findings you documented in questions 1 and 2, what would you do in regard to Patricia Newman's plan of care?

- Click on **Go to the Nurses Station**.
- Click on **Chart**.
- Select the chart for Room **406**.
- Review the **Patient Education** file.
- Review the **Consultations**.

4. Patricia Newman's teaching plan includes a number of different learning objectives, which are similar to expected outcomes. How would you, as the RN, measure the objective/outcome of "patient will comply with dietary recommendations"?

Physical Examination and Vital Signs

👓 **Reading Assignment:** Vital Signs (Chapter 12)
Health Assessment and Physical Examination (Chapter 13)

Patients: Clarence Hughes, Medical-Surgical Floor, Room 404
Patricia Newman, Medical-Surgical Floor, Room 406

Objectives:

- Describe focused physical assessments required based on a patient's medical history findings.
- Recognize abnormal vital signs and physical assessment findings.
- Discuss techniques used to obtain accurate vital signs and physical assessment findings.
- Critique approaches used in the case studies for conducting a physical examination.
- Explain why certain physical examination techniques are used with patients in the case studies.
- Describe focused assessments relevant to changes in a patient's physical condition.
- Discuss how nursing therapies might change vital signs and physical examination findings.

As a nurse, you are responsible for monitoring the condition and progress of your patients so as to anticipate any clinical problems. Valuable sets of tools for assessing a patient's condition include conducting a physical examination and measuring vital signs. Findings from your assessment help to determine the patient's needs and nursing diagnoses and the types of interventions most appropriate. After you administer nursing interventions, physical examination and vital sign measurement also help you to evaluate how the patient responds and determine whether your interventions were successful. The exercises in this lesson will give you a clear sense of how physical examination and vital sign measurement become incorporated into a nurse's routine care and how approaches are individualized based on a patient's history and presenting clinical condition.

Exercise 1

 CD-ROM Activity

 45 minutes

 In this exercise you will visit Clarence Hughes, a 73-year-old African-American male who was admitted to the hospital for a left total knee replacement. You will visit him on his third postop day. You may have worked with Clarence Hughes previously if you already completed Lesson 19.

- Sign in to work at Pacific View Regional Hospital on the Medical-Surgical Floor for Period of Care 1. (*Note:* If you are already in the virtual hospital from a previous exercise, click on **Leave the Floor** and then **Restart the Program** to get to the sign-in window.)
- From the Patient List, select Clarence Hughes (Room 404).
- Click on **Get Report**.
- Click on **Go to Nurses' Station**.
- Click on **Chart**.
- Select the chart for Room **404**.
- Click on and review the **History and Physical**.

1. Clarence Hughes' History and Physical summarizes the condition of his major body systems. For each of the history findings listed below, fill in the physical examination technique(s) you would use to further assess his condition.

History Findings	Physical Examination Techniques
1. Urinary stream is less than it used to be	
2. Smoker for 50 years	
3. Receives pilocarpine drops	
4. Chronic pain in both knees	

2. The clinical report noted that Clarence Hughes feels constipated. List three physical examination techniques you might conduct to assess this problem area further.

3. Clarence Hughes' physical examination findings reveals a Glasgow Coma Scale (GCS) score of 15. This would be interpreted as:
   a. disoriented.
   b. unresponsive.
   c. normal.
   d. hyperactive.

4. True or False. Clarence Hughes' physical examination reveals normal S_1 and S_2 heart sounds. Indicate whether each of the following are true (T) or false (F) in regard to these findings.

   _____ a. S_1 represents the "dub" heard with the stethoscope.

   _____ b. S_2 represents the "dub" heard with the stethoscope.

   _____ c. There is a silent pause between S_1 and S_2.

   _____ d. Normally there is an irregular interval between each sequence of S_1 and S_2.

→ • Click on **Nurse's Notes**.
   • Read the note for Wednesday 0715.

5. The nurse records the following about Clarence Hughes' knee: "may be slightly more swollen than yesterday." There are two approaches you might use to measure the extent of the edema more accurately. Describe each of these approaches.

→ • Click on **Return to Nurses' Station**.
   • Click on **404** to enter Clarence Hughes' room.
   • Review the **Initial Observations.**
   • Click on **Patient Care**.
   • Click on and review the physical assessment findings for the following categories: **Head & Neck, Chest, Abdomen,** and **Lower Extremities**.

6. In the chest assessment, observe the photo of the nurse assessing Clarence Hughes' cardio-vascular function. Place an "X" on the figure below to show at which site the stethoscope was placed to auscultate Clarence Hughes' heart rate.

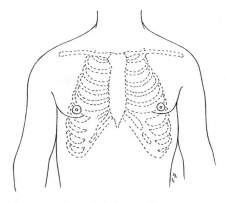

7. Was the nurse using the correct portion of the stethoscope when assessing heart sounds? Give a rationale for your answer.

8. Clarence Hughes' cardiovascular assessment revealed that he had no murmur, click, or rubs. Which portion of the stethoscope do you use to hear murmurs or other extra heart sounds?

9. The examination reveals "impaired sensation in the left leg." Place an X next to all of the following that correctly describe the techniques for assessing sensation.

_____ a. Apply sharp end of a tongue blade to the skin as patient observes.

_____ b. Apply a light stimulus to the skin on both legs.

_____ c. Apply alternately, in a sporadic pattern, both a blunt and sharp end of a tongue blade.

_____ d. Apply sharp stimuli to areas with thicker skin.

_____ e. Apply a light stimulus to the skin as the patient closes the eyes.

10. Explain why the nurse was unable to palpate Clarence Hughes' popliteal pulse in the left leg. What would be another assessment option for the nurse to use?

11. Observe the techniques used by the nurse to examine the patient's abdomen for musculoskeletal function. Was the nurse's technique in the photo correct? Give a rationale.

 • Now click on **Nurse-Client Interactions**.
  • Select and view the video titled **0730: Assessment/Perception of Care**. (*Note:* If this video is not available, check the virtual clock to see whether enough time has elapsed. The video cannot be viewed before its specified time.)
  • Click on **Take Vital Signs**.

12. What factors at the present time would likely cause an increase in Clarence Hughes' heart rate? (Place an X next to all that apply.)

    _____ a. Activity

    _____ b. Pain

    _____ c. Taking medication for constipation

    _____ d. Sitting in bed with head elevated

13. If, when assessing a patient's radial pulse, the rate is irregular, you should count the rate for:
    a. 15 seconds.
    b. 30 seconds.
    c. 1 minute.
    d. 1 minute while another nurse takes an apical pulse.

Exercise 2

 CD-ROM Activity

 30 minutes

 In this exercise you will visit Clarence Hughes, a 73-year-old African-American male who was admitted to the hospital for a left total knee replacement. You will visit him on his third postop day. You may have worked with Clarence Hughes previously if you already completed Exercise 1 or Lesson 19.

  • Sign in to work at Pacific View Regional Hospital on the Medical-Surgical Floor for Period of Care 2. (*Note:* If you are already in the virtual hospital from a previous exercise, click on **Leave the Floor** and then **Restart the Program** to get to the sign-in window.)
  • From the Patient List, select Clarence Hughes (Room 404).
  • Click on **Get Report**.

- Click on **Go to Nurses' Station**.
- Click on **EPR** and **Login**.
- Specify **404** as the patient's room.
- Review the **Vital Signs** record for Clarence Hughes.

1. In the flow chart below, enter Clarence Hughes' vital signs for the designated time periods.

Result	BP	HR	RR	SpO$_2$
Tuesday 1600				
Tuesday 2300				
Wednesday 0715				

2. At this point in time, after reviewing your flow chart, Clarence Hughes' condition can best be described as:
   a. normal and stable.
   b. bradycardic with normal BP, respirations, and oxygen saturation.
   c. hypotensive and bradycardic with normal respirations and oxygen saturation.
   d. low oxygen saturation with hypotension, normal heart rate and respirations.

3. True or False. Pulse oximetry is a reliable indirect measure of oxygen saturation. Indicate whether each of the following descriptions of factors affecting oxygen saturation is true (T) or false (F).

   _____ a. Oxygen saturation would be lowered by an obstruction in the pulmonary capillaries

   _____ b. Oxygen saturation would be lowered by a reduction in hemoglobin

   _____ c. Oxygen saturation would be lowered by build up of edema between the alveoli and pulmonary capillaries

   _____ d. Oxygen saturation would be lowered by a transfusion of red blood cells

- Click on **Exit the EPR**.
- At the Nurses' Station select Room **404** at bottom of screen.
- Review the **Initial Observations.**
- Click on **Patient Care**.
- Click on **Nurse-Client Interactions**.
- Select and view the video titled **1115: Intervention—Airway.** (*Note:* If this video is not available, check the virtual clock to see whether enough time has elapsed. The video cannot be viewed before its specified time.)
- Click on **Take Vital Signs** at the top of the screen.

4. Clarence Hughes is obviously in acute distress. Enter his 1115 vital sign results in the bottom row of the chart below. Then, for comparison purposes, enter his vital signs for the three earlier times listed. (*Note:* You can find these results in the EPR or you can copy your answers from question 1 of this exercise.)

Result	BP	HR	RR	SpO$_2$
Tuesday 1600				
Tuesday 2300				
Wednesday 0715				
Wednesday 1115				

5. Explain the clinical changes occurring for each of Clarence Hughes' vital signs listed in the table above.

   a. Change in BP:

   b. Change in heart rate:

   c. Change in respirations:

   d. Change in SpO$_2$:

6. In measuring vital signs it is important to be accurate. Place an X next to the factors that could cause a false high value in Clarence Hughes' blood pressure.

   _____ a. Loose-fitting cuff

   _____ b. BP cuff too wide

   _____ c. Inflation of BP cuff too slow

   _____ d. Patient's arm above heart level

   _____ e. BP cuff deflated too quickly

7. You are the nurse preparing to examine Clarence Hughes. For the following list of examination categories, which would you identify as priority assessments for this patient?

Head & Neck

_____ Sensory

_____ Mental Status

_____ Thyroid

Chest

_____ Respiratory

_____ Cardiovascular

_____ Integumentary

Upper Extremities

_____ Integumentary

_____ Vascular

Abdomen

_____ Gastrointestinal

_____ Musculoskeletal

Lower Extremities

_____ Vascular

_____ Integumentary

→ • Now, click on **Patient Care**.
  • Review the physical assessment findings for the following categories: Head & Neck (Mental Status), Upper Extremities (Integumentary and Vascular), Chest, and Lower Extremities.

8. Consider what you observed in the interaction and examination data. For each of the findings listed in the left column, match the likely cause in the right column.

Findings	**Cause**
_____ Color in lower extremities pale	a. Anxious and agitated
_____ Attempt to improve ventilation	b. Tachypnea
_____ Pulmonary condition affecting oxygenation	c. Patient sitting up
_____ Reduced oxygen to brain	d. Altered peripheral circulation

➡ • Click on **Chart**.
  • Select the chart for Room **404**.
  • Review the **Physician's Orders**.

9. Explain why the physician ordered an arterial blood gas (ABG).

For questions 10 through 15, fill in the blanks with the appropriate terms describing pulse oximetry.

10. The _____ is an appropriate site for placement of a spring-loaded oximeter probe.

11. Removal of _____ is necessary to ensure proper light transmission when using an oximeter.

12. The pulse wave on the oximeter will be _____ by peripheral edema.

13. Normally, when first applying an oximeter probe, it takes _____ to _____ seconds for a reading to appear.

➡ • Click on **Return to Room 404**.
  • Click on **Leave the Floor**.
  • Click on **Restart the Program**.
  • Sign in to work at Pacific View Regional Hospital on the Medical-Surgical Floor for Period of Care 3. (*Note:* If you are already in the virtual hospital from a previous exercise, click on **Leave the Floor** and then **Restart the Program** to get to the sign-in window.)
  • From the Patient List, select Clarence Hughes (Room 404) and click on **Get Report**.
  • Review the clinical report.
  • Click on **Go to Nurses' Station**.

14. Clarence Hughes was experiencing a pulmonary embolus. An embolus blocks blood flow in an artery supplying blood to the lung. In this case the embolus probably originated in the patient's popliteal vein, where tests have shown a thrombus is located. Which of the following are signs of venous insufficiency? (Place an X next to all that apply.)

_____ a. Absent pulse

_____ b. Marked edema

_____ c. Cyanosis of the skin

_____ d. Normal pulse

_____ e. Shiny skin

Exercise 3

 CD-ROM Activity

 30 minutes

Patricia Newman is a 61-year-old Caucasian female with a history of emphysema for 12 years. She has been admitted to the emergency department in moderate respiratory distress. You may have worked with Patricia Newman previously if you completed Lesson 2, 3, 9, or 10.

• Sign in to work at Pacific View Regional Hospital on the Medical-Surgical Floor for Period of Care 1. (*Note:* If you are already in the virtual hospital from a previous exercise, click on **Leave the Floor** and then **Restart the Program** to get to the sign-in window.)
• From the Patient List, select Patricia Newman (Room 406).
• Click on **Get Report**.

1. Match the vital sign findings on the left with the correct terminology on the right.

Vital Signs	**Terminology**
_____ 168/94	a. Tachypneic
_____ 112	b. Hypertensive
_____ 32	c. Febrile
_____ 102° F	d. Tachycardic

 • Click on **Go to Nurses' Station**.
• Click on **Chart**.
• Select the chart for Room **406**.
• Click on and review the **History and Physical**.

2. Patricia Newman has a history of emphysema and hypertension. What is one factor in her history that could be associated with both conditions?

3. Patricia Newman's physical examination reveals coarse crackles throughout the lung fields. In the list below and on the next page, place an X next to all entries that correctly describe the features of crackles.

_____ a. Heard over anterior lateral lung field

_____ b. Best heard in dependent lobes

_____ c. Primarily heard over trachea and bronchi

_____ d. Caused by high-velocity air flow

_____ e. Result of inflamed pleura

_____ f. Result of sudden reinflation of alveoli

_____ g. High-pitched, fine and short sound

_____ h. Dry grating sound

_____ i. Low-pitched rumbling sound

 • Click on **Return to Nurses' Station**.
• Click on **406** to go to Patricia Newman's room.
• Review the **Initial Observations.**
• Click on **Patient Care**.
• Select the **Nurse-Client Interactions**.
• Select and view the video titled **0730: Prioritizing Interventions**. (*Note:* If this video is not available, check the virtual clock to see whether enough time has elapsed. The video cannot be viewed before its specified time.)
• Click on **Physical Assessment**.
• Click on **Chest** and observe the complete examination of the chest.

  4. The respiratory assessment of the chest notes Patricia Newman's breathing is labored and shallow. What assessment techniques are used to determine these findings?

  5. Again, observe the nurse as she performs the respiratory assessment of the chest. In the diagram below, mark a "1" in the circle where the stethoscope is placed by the nurse. Then trace the next steps that would be used to assess the lungs anteriorly (assuming the nurse has followed the correct sequence so far).

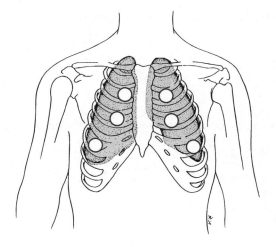

 • Now click on **Back & Spine** and then on **Respiratory**.

6. Observe the respiratory assessment findings for the back and spine. The findings note that Patricia Newman has hyperessonance to percussion. Explain the reason for this finding.

→ • Click on **Take Vital Signs** at the top of the screen.

7. Match the blood pressure type on the left with the correct auscultatory sound on the right.

Blood Pressure Type	**Auscultatory Sound**
_____ Systolic pressure	a. First Korotkoff sound
_____ Diastolic pressure	b. Second Korotkoff sound
	c. Third Korotkoff sound
	d. Fourth Korotkoff sound
	e. Fifth Korotkoff sound

8. Because Patricia Newman is hypertensive, she is at risk for presenting an auscultatory gap during blood pressure measurement.

a. What is an auscultatory gap?

b. It typically occurs between which heart sounds?

c. How do you avoid an auscultatory gap when measuring BP?

Communication with the Patient and the Health Care Team

/Oᴼᴼᴼᴼᴼᴼᴼᴼᴼᴼᴼᴼᴼᴼᴼᴼᴼᴼᴼᴼᴼᴼᴼᴼᴼᴼᴼᴼᴼ

Reading Assignment: Communication (Chapter 9)

Patients: Dorothy Grant, Obstetrics Floor, Room 201
                  Kathryn Doyle, Skilled Nursing Floor, Room 503

Objectives:

- Discuss perceptions of communication interactions viewed in the case studies.
- Describe levels of communication.
- Identify forms of communication viewed in the case studies.
- Describe elements of professional communication.
- Identify factors that create barriers to communication.
- Identify therapeutic communication techniques.

At the core of nursing are the caring relationships formed between nurses and patients. All of our behavior communicates, and all communication influences the behavior of others. Communication is the means for establishing therapeutic relationships with patients. The ability to communicate effectively helps you to establish the important connection that allows you to deliver quality care to patients.

Talking *with* patients, not *at* patients, can be difficult. The same is true in regard to patients' families. Communication requires sensitivity, active participation, and an astute interpretation of what people convey through their words and behavior. You must be willing to know a patient and to reveal a bit of yourself in order to establish the trust and confidence necessary to communicate therapeutically.

Exercise 1

 CD-ROM Activity

 45 minutes

 In this exercise you will visit Dorothy Grant, a pregnant 25-year-old who was admitted to the hospital after blunt trauma to the abdomen. You may have worked with Dorothy Grant previously if you already completed Lesson 18.

- Sign in to work at Pacific View Regional Hospital on the Obstetrics Floor for Period of Care 2. (*Note:* If you are already in the virtual hospital from a previous exercise, click on **Leave the Floor** and then **Restart the Program** to get to the sign-in window.)
- From the Patient List, select Dorothy Grant (Room 201).
- Click on **Get Report**.
- Click on **Go to Nurses' Station**.
- Click on **Chart**.
- Select the chart for Room **201**.
- Click on and review the **Nursing Admission**.

1. The report tells you that the patient has been anxious and crying. As you prepare to go to Dorothy Grant's room to meet her, what might you consider doing in your initial communication approach? Describe in detail.

2. Active listening will be an important communication technique as you talk with Dorothy Grant. There are several nonverbal skills that facilitate attentive listening. Complete the descriptions for the acronym SOLER below.

   S

   O

   L

   E

   R

 - Click on **Return to Nurses' Station**.
- Click on Room **201** at bottom of screen.
- Review the **Initial Observations**.
- Click on **Patient Care**.
- Click on **Nurse-Client Interactions**.
- Select and view the video titled **1115: Nurse-Patient Communication**. (*Note:* If this video is not available, check the virtual clock to see whether enough time has elapsed. The video cannot be viewed before its specified time.)

3. The nurse opens the conversation by asking, "Would you like to talk about your concerns?"

   a. What type of question is this?

   b. Was this the most appropriate way to begin the conversation? If not, how would you restate the question?

→ • Observe the video interaction once more.

4. As you observe the nurse interact with Dorothy Grant, select the listening techniques the nurse used from the list below. (Place an X next to all that apply.)

   _____ a. Sit facing patient

   _____ b. Use an open posture

   _____ c. Lean toward patient

   _____ d. Establish/maintain eye contact

   _____ e. Relax

5. During the video, the nurse says to the patient, "Right now, your first priority is your well-being and the well-being of your baby." This is an example of what therapeutic technique?
   a. Empathy
   b. Sharing hope
   c. Providing information
   d. Paraphrasing

6. Dorothy Grant expresses how valuable her sister has been as a resource, but states that her parents "act like nothing is going on."

   a. The nurse responds, "That must be so frustrating." What type of communication technique is this?

   b. What is the patient's response to this technique?

7. What communication and caring technique does the nurse use to initially focus on the importance of monitoring Dorothy Grant's obstetric condition? What is the purpose of this technique?

→ • Observe the video interaction one final time.

8. Complete the categories listed below by describing Dorothy Grant's nonverbal behaviors for each category.

Personal appearance

Facial expression

Eye contact

Gestures

Sounds

9. As the nurse interacts with Dorothy Grant, she is assuming which zone of personal space?
   a. Public zone
   b. Personal zone
   c. Intimate zone
   d. Social zone

Exercise 2

 CD-ROM Activity

 30 minutes

 In this exercise you will visit Kathryn Doyle, a 79-year-old Caucasian female who was admitted following a "fall" at home in which she sustained a left hip fracture. You may have worked with Kathryn Doyle previously if you already completed Lesson 4, 6, 7, 8, or 12.

- Sign in to work at Pacific View Regional Hospital on the Skilled Nursing Floor for Period of Care 1. (*Note:* If you are already in the virtual hospital from a previous exercise, click on **Leave the Floor** and then **Restart the Program** to get to the sign-in window.)
- From the Patient List, select Kathryn Doyle (Room 503).
- Click on **Get Report**.
- Click on **Go to Nurses' Station**.
- Click on **Chart**.
- Select the chart for Room **503**.
- Review the patient's **History and Physical**.
- Next, review the **Nursing Admission**, paying particular attention to Self-Perception and Role Relationships.
- Click on **Return to Nurses' Station**.
- Click on Room **503** at the bottom of the screen.
- Review the **Initial Observations**.
- Click on **Patient Care**.
- Click on **Nurse-Client Interactions**.
- Select and view the video titled **0730: Assessment—Biopsychosocial**. (*Note:* If this video is not available, check the virtual clock to see whether enough time has elapsed. The video cannot be viewed before its specified time.)

1. After reviewing data from the H&P and Nursing Admission, you know that Kathryn Doyle has concerns about returning home. In the video interaction between the nurse and patient, what nonverbal behavior did Kathryn Doyle display in each of the following categories?

Voice tone

Facial expression

Eye contact

2. List three characteristics of eye contact.

➡ • Observe the same video once again.

3. Kathryn Doyle stated, "I just don't feel like myself." The nurse responded, "Do you have any concerns you would like to talk about?" Was the nurse's response appropriate? Explain.

4. Kathryn Doyle explains, "Well, I've been thinking of going home and wondering just what it's going to be like." For each of the communication techniques listed below, write an appropriate response to learn more about her feelings toward going home.

Paraphrasing

Sharing observation

Clarifying

➡ • Now, select and view the video titled **0733: Planning—Fact Finding**. (*Note:* If this video is not available, check the virtual clock to see whether enough time has elapsed. The video cannot be viewed before its specified time.)

5. The nurse responds, "Oh, why do you think that is?" What type of response is this?
   a. Asking for explanation
   b. Clarifying
   c. Focusing
   d. Automatic response

6. What would have been a better response on the part of the nurse?

7. Match the phrase on the right with the nontherapeutic communication technique on the left.

Technique	Phrase
_____ Automatic response	a. "You shouldn't stop eating. It will make it difficult for your hip to heal."
_____ False reassurance	b. "Sons just do not understand their mothers."
_____ Disapproval	c. "Don't be concerned. Your weight loss is not a problem."
_____ Sympathy	d. "I'm sorry about your husband. It must be such a heavy burden for you."

8. List five principles needed for professional communication.

9. By using assertive behavior, a nurse has the advantage of conveying the ability to:
   a. empathize.
   b. make decisions.
   c. judge others' behavior.
   d. depend on others for agreement.

Patient Education in Practice

Reading Assignment: Client Education (Chapter 10)

Patient: Patricia Newman, Medical-Surgical Floor, Room 406

Objectives:

- Identify purposes of patient education.
- Describe basic learning principles.
- Assess the learning needs of a case study patient.
- Apply critical thinking in planning a teaching plan for a case study patient.
- Describe domains of learning to include in a patient's plan of care.
- Discuss factors to consider in designing a teaching plan.
- Identify factors that influence a patient's readiness to learn.
- Write learning objectives for a teaching plan.
- Discuss teaching methods appropriate to select case study patients.
- Identify approaches for evaluating learning.

It is your responsibility as a nurse to provide patient education so that patients and families are able to make informed decisions about their health and to assume self-care activities. Patient education is one of your most important roles as a nurse. Your challenge is to develop the best teaching plan that matches the patient's learning needs and ability to learn with relevant and appropriate teaching strategies. Because most patients continue health care activities in the home, you must be aware of all of the educational resources available to ensure a smooth and safe transition of care. Evaluation of patient learning is also critical to ensure that patients have obtained necessary knowledge and the ability to perform self-care activities.

Exercise 1

  CD-ROM Activity

 45 minutes

In this exercise you will visit Patricia Newman, a 61-year-old Caucasian female who has a history of emphysema, osteoporosis, and hypertension. She has been admitted to the hospital in moderate respiratory distress. You may have worked with Patricia Newman previously if you already completed Lesson 2, 3, 9, or 10.

- Sign in to work at Pacific View Regional Hospital on the Medical-Surgical Floor for Period of Care 1. (*Note:* If you are already in the virtual hospital from a previous exercise, click on **Leave the Floor** and then **Restart the Program** to get to the sign-in window.)
- From the Patient List, select Patricia Newman (Room 406).
- Click on **Get Report**.
- Click on **Go to Nurses' Station**.
- Click on **Chart**.
- Select the chart for Room **406**.
- Review the **Nursing Admission**.

1. Using data from the Nursing Admission, consider each of the following learning principles and describe how they apply to Patricia Newman. Be specific.

Attention set

Compliance

Psychosocial adaptation to illness

Physical capability

2. What behavior increases Patricia Newman's risk for worsening emphysema?
   a. Not getting a flu shot
   b. Family history of lung disease
   c. Smoking cigarettes
   d. Becoming underweight

 • Review the **Physician's Orders**. (*Study Tip:* Review the type and purpose of all medications ordered in your pharmacology text.)

• Click on **Consultations** and review the consult notes.

3. Based on the information you have reviewed so far, list four learning needs that apply to Patricia Newman.

4. Considering Patricia Newman's learning needs, match the learning domains with the learning needs below.

Learning Need	Learning Domain
_____ Adopting health promotion behaviors (e.g., routine breast exams)	a. Cognitive
	b. Affective
_____ Understanding the benefits achieved from not smoking	c. Psychomotor
_____ Manipulation of a metered-dose inhaler	
_____ Being able to count caloric intake each day	

 • Click on **Return to the Nurses' Station**.
• Click on to Room **406** at the bottom of the screen.
• Review the **Initial Observations.**
• Select **Patient Care**.
• Click on **Nurse-Client Interactions**.
• Select and view the videos titled **0730: Prioritizing Interventions** and **0740: Evaluation—Response to Care**. (*Note:* If either video is not available, check the virtual clock to see whether enough time has elapsed. The videos cannot be viewed before their specified time.)

5. The respiratory therapist will be working with Patricia Newman on use of a peak flow meter as a means to detect changes in her airway resistance. Place an X next to each of the following factors that should be assessed in relation to Patricia Newman's ability to learn.

_____ a. Distractors in the room during demonstration of meter

_____ b. Coordination and endurance to hold meter and perform breathing maneuver

_____ c. Patient's belief in need to improve lung function

_____ d. Patient's learning style preference

6. As Patricia Newman's nurse, you identify the nursing diagnosis of Deficient Knowledge regarding use of peak flow meter related to lack of exposure to information. You collaborate with the respiratory therapist to develop a teaching plan for Patricia Newman so that she can use the meter routinely at home. Complete the following critical thinking diagram for planning by writing the letter of each critical thinking factor under its proper category.

Knowledge

1. _____

2. _____

Experience　　　　**PLANNING**　　　　**Standards**

3. _____　　　　　　　　　　4. _____

　　　　　　　　　　　　　　　　　　　5. _____

Attitudes

6. _____

Critical Thinking Factors

a. Be creative in planning to have neighbor attend teaching session so that patient will have a coach to reinforce meter technique.
b. Review information regarding the effects emphysema has on peak flow rate.
c. Consider how you have instructed patients in the past on use of medical devices.
d. Review manufacturer's directions for proper use of flow meter.
e. Individualize teaching sessions to plan for frequent rest periods and reinforcement.
f. Consider learning principles that influence patient's motivation.

7. Write a learning objective for teaching Patricia Newman on the use of a peak flow meter.

• Click on **Chart**.
  • Select the chart for Room **406**.
  • Review the **Patient Education** file.

8. For each of the learning goals listed on Patricia Newman's teaching plan, critique and explain how the goal or objective should be written more clearly.

    a. Patient will comply with dietary recommendations:

    b. Patient will understand rationale and perform pursed-lip breathing:

    c. Patient will demonstrate correct use of MDI:

9. When instructing Patricia Newman on the use of the peak flow meter, demonstration should be combined with discussion. What might you include in the discussion?

 • Click on **Return to Room 406**.
  • Click on **Patient Care**.
  • Select **Nurse-Client Interactions**.
  • Select and view the video titled **0750: Evaluation—Patient Teaching**. (*Note:* If this video is not available, check the virtual clock to see whether enough time has elapsed. The video cannot be viewed before its specified time.)

10. During the interaction, the nurse missed an opportunity to evaluate Patricia Newman's learning. What should the nurse have done?

Exercise 2

 CD-ROM Activity

30 minutes

In this exercise you will visit Patricia Newman, a 61-year-old Caucasian female who has a history of emphysema, osteoporosis, and hypertension. She has been admitted to the hospital in moderate respiratory distress. You may have worked with Patricia Newman previously if you already completed Exercise 1 or Lesson 2, 3, 9, or 10.

- Sign in to work at Pacific View Regional Hospital on the Medical-Surgical Floor for Period of Care 2 (*Note:* If you are already in the virtual hospital from a previous exercise, click on **Leave the Floor** and then **Restart the Program** to get to the sign-in window.)
- From the Patient List, select Patricia Newman (Room 406).
- Click on **Get Report**.
- Click on **Go to Nurses' Station**.
- Click on **Chart**.
- Select the chart for Room **406**.
- Review the **Nursing Admission**.
- Review the **Physician's Orders**.

1. There are three primary purposes of patient education. Match the following education topics with the purpose applicable to Patricia Newman.

Purpose	Education Topic
_____ Health promotion	a. Walking more frequently at longer intervals
_____ Health restoration	b. Quitting Smoking
_____ Coping with impaired function	c. Purpose and schedule of inhaler
	d. Purpose of flu shots
	e. Administration of home oxygen

- Click on **Return to Nurses' Station**.
- Select Room **406** at the bottom of the screen.
- Review the **Initial Observations.**
- Click on **Patient Care.**
- Select **Nurse-Client Interactions**.
- Select and view the video titled **1100: Care Coordination**. (*Note:* If this video is not available, check the virtual clock to see whether enough time has elapsed. The video cannot be viewed before its specified time.)

2. Patricia Newman's statement, "I know I should quit smoking" is an example of which learning principle?
   a. Ability to learn
   b. A learning need
   c. Motivation
   d. Compliance

True or False. Select true or false for questions 3 through 7.

3. Patients who are highly anxious will often be motivated to learn.
   a. True
   b. False

4. Patients learn better when you build on their existing level of knowledge.
   a. True
   b. False

5. Patients who are in pain often have an impaired ability to learn.
   a. True
   b. False

6. Assessing whether a patient is able to convert food portions to calories and add total calories determines an ability to learn.
   a. True
   b. False

7. A patient who grieves over the loss of physical function will most likely learn about long-range health restrictions during the phase of bargaining.
   a. True
   b. False

8. The physician ordered Patricia Newman to self-administer ipratropium bromide by metered-dose inhaler. Based on her admission data, what aspect of this activity might be difficult for the patient to perform? (*Study Tip:* Review skill for using metered-dose inhaler on pages 382-385 in your textbook.)
   a. Reading the medication label
   b. Understanding the directions
   c. Depressing the medication canister
   d. Sitting up to inhale the medication

 • Click on **Chart**.
   • Select the chart for Room **406**.
   • Review the **Patient Education** file.

9. Patricia Newman will be receiving instruction on a number of topics. Match each of the following teaching topics with the appropriate instructional method.

Instructional Method	**Teaching Topic**
_____ Simulation	a. Pursed-lip breathing
_____ Demonstration	b. Side effects of medications
_____ Role playing	c. Planning a dinner high in protein
_____ One-to-one discussion	d. Learning to say no when a friend offers a cigarette
_____ Use of analogies	e. Explaining how high blood pressure creates an effect similar to forcing water through a constricted hose.

10. For each of the instructional topics listed below, identify the correct evaluation method.

Self-administration of a metered-dose inhaler

Patient's ability to increase distance walking

Patient's compliance with a high-caloric diet

Documentation Principles

🕮 **Reading Assignment:** Documentation and Reporting (Chapter 8)

Patients: Kathryn Doyle, Skilled Nursing Floor, Room 503
Pablo Rodriguez, Medical-Surgical Floor, Room 405

Objectives:

- Identify the purpose of medical records.
- Identify elements of quality documentation in written records and verbal reports.
- Apply use of military time in recording.
- Write a nursing progress note.
- Explain the purpose of flow charting.
- Critique the quality of a change-of-shift report.
- Describe elements of a telephone order.
- Explain the type of information to communicate when a patient's condition changes.

Recording and reporting are two skills that must be performed accurately and in a timely and effective manner. The quality of your nursing care depends on your ability to communicate with other nurses and members of the health care team. All health care providers must know their patients, the problems they develop, their progress, and their response to treatments. Excellent documentation and reporting of information ensures that you have the knowledge you need about patients to provide continuity of care from shift to shift or visit to visit. In order for you to become competent in documentation, you must follow both legal and regulatory standards for how and what to record about your patients' care.

Exercise 1

 CD-ROM Activity

 45 minutes

 In this exercise you will visit Kathryn Doyle, a 79-year-old Caucasian female who entered the skilled nursing unit after repair of an intertrochanteric fracture 2 weeks ago. You may have worked with Kathryn Doyle previously if you already completed Lesson 4, 7, or 12.

- Sign in to work at Pacific View Regional Hospital on the Skilled Nursing Floor for Period of Care 1. (*Note:* If you are already in the virtual hospital from a previous exercise, click on **Leave the Floor** and then **Restart the Program** to get to the sign-in window.)
- From the Patient List, select Kathryn Doyle (Room 503).
- Click on **Get Report**.

1. After reviewing the report summary, list two examples of inaccurate information given in the report.

2. The report summary notes that Kathryn Doyle received oxycodone and acetaminophen for pain in the left hip. Place an X next to each of the following criteria that should have been included in the description of pain.

_____ a. Condition of right hip

_____ b. Onset of pain

_____ c. Severity of pain

_____ d. Action of pain medication

_____ e. Factors that worsen pain

_____ f. Duration of pain

- Click on **Go to Nurses' Station**.
- Click on **Chart**.
- Select the chart for Room **503**.
- Review the **Nurse's Notes** for Wednesday at 0715.
- Now, click on **Return to Nurses' Station**.
- Access the EPR by clicking on the computer screen on the counter or clicking on **EPR** at the top of your screen.
- Click on **Login**.
- Select Room **503** and review the **Vital Signs**.

3. Although the nurse's note reported Kathryn Doyle to have a low-grade fever, more accurate information was available in the EPR. What was Kathryn Doyle's actual temperature?

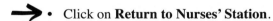 • Review the other entries on the Vital Signs flow sheet.

4. List two advantages of a flow sheet.

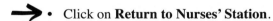 • Click on **Return to Nurses' Station**.
  • Click on **Chart**.
  • Select the chart for Room **503**.
  • Review the **Nurse's Notes** for 0555.

5. The entry of 0555 represents what time in standard time?
   a. 5:55 p.m.
   b. 12:05 a.m.
   c. 5:55 a.m.
   d. 12:55 p.m.

6. The nurse's entry of "States she 'could not get comfortable'" is an example of which documentation characteristic?
   a. Accuracy
   b. Complete
   c. Factual
   d. Current

7. Rewrite the narrative note for 0555 in a PIE format below.

   P

   I

   E

8. How might the nurse have made the 0555 narrative note more complete in regard to Kathryn Doyle's problem of pain management?

➤ • Still in the chart, review the **Nurse's Notes** for Tuesday at 1825.
 • Next, go to the **Physician's Orders** and review the entry for Tuesday at 1530.

9. The nurse's note for 1825 refers to a TO verified.

 a. Does the nurse's signature on this note verify the telephone order?

 b. Is the nurse's signature the correct way for signing off a note? If not, explain.

10. Is the physician's order for the psych consult completed correctly? Explain.

➤ • Click on **Nursing Admission** and review the summary.

11. Medical records serve several purposes. Match each application of information from Kathryn Doyle's record with its purpose.

Application	Purpose
_____ Data show that Kathryn Doyle's allergy history was entered.	a. Communication of patient problem
_____ A review of Kathryn Doyle's self-perception helps demonstrate factors that influence a person's body image.	b. Use of records to research characteristics of patients who have hip surgery
_____ Kathryn Doyle's assessment shows she is sleeping poorly, tires easily, and receives no regular exercise.	c. Auditing of chart for regulatory requirements
_____ Kathryn Doyle is age 79. She has a history of osteoporosis, she fell at home, and she takes calcium daily.	d. Education for understanding nature of nursing concepts

Exercise 2

  CD-ROM Activity

 30 minutes

In this exercise you will visit Pablo Rodriguez, a 71-year-old Hispanic male who is suffering from advanced non-small-cell lung carcinoma. You may have worked with Pablo Rodriguez previously if you already completed Lesson 12, 13, or 19.

- Sign in to work at Pacific View Regional Hospital on the Medical-Surgical Floor for Period of Care 1. (*Note:* If you are already in the virtual hospital from a previous exercise, click on **Leave the Floor** and then **Restart the Program** to get to the sign-in window.)
- From the Patient List, select Pablo Rodriguez (Room 405).
- Click on **Get Report**.

1. This report summary is an example of the information typically shared between nurses during change-of-shift report. One of the advantages of oral reports is the ability to ask questions. After reviewing Pablo Rodriguez's report, list three questions you might ask the night nurse.

True or False. Select true or false for questions 2 through 6.

2. When giving a report, it is most important to be complete, so take whatever time is needed.
   a. True
   b. False

3. One of the best forms of report is to read information from the patient's Kardex.
   a. True
   b. False

4. When giving a transfer report, include a discussion of any assessments that should be completed shortly after transfer.
   a. True
   b. False

5. Whenever you take a telephone report, repeat the entire report to ensure accuracy.
   a. True
   b. False

6. Telephone orders and verbal orders need to be cosigned by the ordering physician, usually within 24 hours.
   a. True
   b. False

7. For each of the actions listed below, write "Do" if it correctly applies to the change-of-shift report or "Don't" if it does not apply to the change-of shift report.

a. Describe the basic steps of how the patient uses a PCA.

b. Describe objective measures such as oxygen at 3 liters.

c. Evaluate result of morphine when given for pain in nodules.

d. Review the patient's age, occupation, and education.

e. Identify and explain the patient's immediate priorities of care.

 • Click on **Go to Nurses' Station**.
• Click on Room **405** at the bottom of the screen.
• Review the **Initial Observations.**
• Click on **Patient Care**.
• Click on **Nurse-Client Interactions**.
• Select and view the video titled **0735: Patient Perceptions**. (*Note:* If this video is not available, check the virtual clock to see whether enough time has elapsed. The video cannot be viewed before its specified time.)

8. Observe and listen to the video several times. Now pretend you are the nurse in the video and write a DAR note below that describes the interaction with Pablo Rodriguez.

D

A

R

 • Click on **Return to Nurses' Station**.
• Click on **Chart**.
• Select the chart for Room **405**.
• Read the **Nurse's Notes**.

9. The note states "0700 IV bolus of morphine sulfate 6 mg given as ordered." This is an example of which guideline for recording?
a. Completeness
b. Organized
c. Current
d. Focused

Fill in the blanks to complete the following legal guidelines for recording.

10. Do not leave a _____ _____ in a narrative note because another person could add incorrect information there.

11. All entries in a chart should be _____ to prevent misinterpretation of information.

12. Correct any _____ promptly to avoid a negative outcome for the patient.

13. When an error has been made in recording, correct it by drawing a _____ through the error.

14. Always chart only for _____ to ensure accountability for information in the record.

15. For each of the following standard times, write the correct military time.

    6:23 a.m.

    7:10 p.m.

    12:05 a.m.

    11:55 p.m.

LESSON 7

Safe Medication Administration in Practice

Reading Assignment: Administering Medications (Chapter 14)

Patients: Piya Jordan, Medical-Surgical Floor, Room 403
Kathryn Doyle, Skilled Nursing Floor, Room 503

Objectives:

- Discuss the rationale for medications ordered for patients in the case studies.
- Explain how to apply the 6 rights of medication administration.
- Perform medication dosage calculations.
- Explain nursing implications for administering medications.
- Describe potential sources of medication errors.
- Identify factors that influence selection of form and route of a medication for administration.
- Discuss factors in the case studies that would contraindicate administration of a medication.
- Correctly describe steps for administering a medication.

Medication administration is one of the more important responsibilities of a professional nurse because of the risks involved. Any given medication has the potential for creating harmful effects if administered inappropriately or incorrectly. The busy health care environment poses many barriers to safe medication administration. Thus it is important to learn how to attend to the preparation and administration of medications. You can never be too cautious in administering medications. Always follow the 6 rights of drug administration and be aware of the principles used to calculate and prepare medications safely and accurately. Know the effects that medications may have on your patient's behavior and physical condition so that you can properly monitor the patient and evaluate whether the drugs have been effective.

Patient education is an important part of drug therapy. Patients must obtain the necessary information to self-administer medications safely and know how to monitor their response to medications. Home environments and daily routines influence how patients take their medications. It is important to problem-solve with patients and families to anticipate possible barriers to safe medication administration in the home and workplace.

Exercise 1

  CD-ROM Activity

 45 minutes

In this exercise you will visit Piya Jordan, a 68-year-old Asian-American female who entered the hospital after an emergency department admission for abdominal pain, nausea, and vomiting. She underwent abdominal surgery for the removal of a mass in her right lower quadrant. You may have worked with Piya Jordan previously if you already completed Lesson 10, 14, or 15.

- Sign in to work at Pacific View Regional Hospital on the Medical-Surgical Floor for Period of Care 1. (*Note:* If you are already in the virtual hospital from a previous exercise, click on **Leave the Floor** and then **Restart the Program** to get to the sign-in window.)
- From the Patient List, select Piya Jordan (Room 403).
- Click on **Get Report**.
- Click on **Go to Nurses' Station**.
- Click on **Chart**.
- Select the chart for Room **403**.
- Review the **History and Physical**.
- Next, review the **Physician's Orders** for Tuesday and Wednesday mornings.

1. Piya Jordan has orders for a number of medications postoperatively. Match each medication listed below with the rationale for its administration.

Medication	Rationale
_____ Digoxin 0.125 mg IV	a. Reduce fever
_____ Famotidine 20 mg IV	b. Reduce gastric acid secretion
_____ Cefotetan 1 g IV	c. Slow the heart rate of atrial fibrillation
_____ Acetaminophen 650 mg per rectum q6h	d. Prevent postop wound infection

2. Review the physician's postop medication orders once again. Are there any dangerous abbreviations used? If so, what is the preferred alternative?

- Once again, review the physician's medication orders for Piya Jordan.
- Now click on **Return to Nurses' Station**.
- Click on the **Medication Room**.
- Select the **MAR** and click tab **403**.
- Review the MAR for drugs due to be given Wednesday between 0730 and 0815.

3. Place an X next to all of the following statements that describe activities for correctly following the 6 rights of medication administration.

_____ a. Compare MAR with physician's written order for the name of a medication.

_____ b. Review the patient record for the patient's allergies.

_____ c. Review the supply cart for the size of syringes.

_____ d. Check the MAR against the physician's written order for the route to give a medication.

_____ e. Compare the physician's written order for a medication with the times selected on the MAR for scheduled administration.

➡ • Click on **Return to Medication Room**.
  • Based on your care for Piya Jordan, access the various storage areas of the Medication Room to obtain the necessary medications you need to administer.
  • For each area you access, select the medication you plan to administer and then click **Put Medication on Tray**. When finished with a storage area, click on **Close Drawer** or **Close Bin**.
  • Click **View Medication Room**.
  • Now click on **Preparation** and choose the correct medication to administer. Click **Prepare**.
  • Click **Next** and choose the correct patient to administer this medication to. Click **Finish**.
  • You can **Review Your Medications** and then **Return to Medication Room** when ready.

4. How much of the digoxin did you prepare in a syringe for Piya Jordan?

5. Which of the following medications did you prepare for this time period? (Place an X next to all that apply.)

_____ a. Enoxaparin 40 mg

_____ b. KCl 20 mEq in 250 mL NS

_____ c. Digoxin 0.125 mg

_____ d. Morphine sulfate 2.5 mg per 1 mL

_____ e. Cefotetan 1 g

- Click on **Return to Nurses' Station**.
- Click on Room **403** at the bottom of the screen.
- Click on **Patient Care**.
- Click on **Medication Administration**.

6. Before administering digoxin to Piya Jordan, what should you assess?
   a. Blood pressure and IV infusion
   b. Apical heart rate and IV infusion
   c. Potassium level and blood pressure
   d. Patient's level of discomfort and range of motion in knees

7. Before administering the digoxin, what is the main function of the IV infusion you should assess?

- Perform any necessary assessments and assess any pertinent information before administering your medications.
- After you have collected the appropriate assessment data and are ready for administration, click **Patient Care** and **Medication Administration**. Verify that the correct patient and medication(s) appear in the left-hand window. Then click the down arrow next to Select. From the drop-down menu, select **Administer** and complete the Administration Wizard by providing any information requested. When the Wizard stops asking for information, click **Administer to Patient**. Specify **Yes** when asked whether this administration should be recorded in the MAR. Finally, click **Finish**.

True or False. Select true or false for questions 8 through 11.

8. IV administration of digoxin creates a greater risk to the patient than IV administration of KCl.
   a. True
   b. False

9. After choosing to hold cefotetan because of Piya Jordan's allergy, you should contact the prescriber immediately.
   a. True
   b. False

10. When you are administering a medication by an intermittent infusion, turn off the main IV infusion as the medication is infused.
    a. True
    b. False

11. After administering an intermittent infusion, you should discard the bag of medication and the IV tubing.
    a. True
    b. False

12. Why is Piya Jordan not given her digoxin by mouth?

Exercise 2

 CD-ROM Activity

 45 minutes

 In this exercise you will visit Piya Jordan, a 68-year-old Asian-American female who entered the hospital after an emergency department admission for abdominal pain, nausea, and vomiting. She underwent abdominal surgery for the removal of a mass in her right lower quadrant. You may have worked with Piya Jordan previously if you already completed Exercise 1 or Lesson 7, 10, 12, 14, or 15.

- Sign in to work at Pacific View Regional Hospital on the Medical-Surgical Floor for Period of Care 2. (*Note:* If you are already in the virtual hospital from a previous exercise, click on **Leave the Floor** and then **Restart the Program** to get to the sign-in window.)
- From the Patient List, select Piya Jordan (Room 403).
- Click on **Get Report**.
- Click on **Go to Nurses' Station**.
- Click on **Chart**.
- Select the chart for Room **403**.
- Review the **History and Physical**.
- Then select **Nurse's Notes** and review.
- Next, review the **Physician's Orders**.

1. The physician ordered ondansetron 4 mg IV q6h PRN for nausea. Which of the following statements are true about a PRN order?

_____ a. It calls for a single dose of a medication to be given only once.

_____ b. It is a type of order that requires the medication to be given at a specific time.

_____ c. It is an order prescribed for a time when a patient requires it.

_____ d. It is the only type of order canceled when a patient goes to surgery.

The physician also ordered enoxaparin 40 mg subQ. Fill in the blanks below to describe principles for administering subcutaneous injections.

2. A subcutaneous injection requires a _____ gauge needle.

3. A _____ to _____ ml syringe is usually adequate for a subcutaneous injection.

4. The best site for administering heparin is the _____.

5. Injecting heparin slowly over 30 seconds may create less _____.

6. Considering Piya Jordan's physical build, what needle length and angle of insertion would you use for the enoxaparin injection?

- Click on **Return to Nurses' Station**.
- Click on Room **403** at the bottom of the screen.
- Review the **Initial Observations**.
- Click on **Patient Care**.
- Click on **Nurse-Client Interactions**.
- Select and view the video titled **1115: Interventions—Nausea, Blood**. (*Note:* If this video is not available, check the virtual clock to see whether enough time has elapsed. The video cannot be viewed before its specified time.)
- Next, click on **Take Vital Signs** at the top of the screen.

7. After reviewing the physician's medication orders and the nurse-client interaction, is it appropriate to administer the ordered acetaminophen for Piya Jordan? Explain.

8. Piya Jordan has complained of nausea. Go to the Medication Room to prepare ondansetron and answer the following questions.

   a. The ondansetron comes in a vial/ampule containing how many mL?

   b. What is the correct volume of ondansetron to administer?

- Click on **Patient Care**.
- Click on **Physical Assessment**.

9. What body system would you assess prior to administering the ondansetron? Explain your answer.

• Click on **Medication Room**.

- Click on **MAR** to determine the medications that Piya Jordan is ordered to receive. (*Note:* You may click on **Review MAR** at any time to verify correct medication order. Remember to look at the patient name on the MAR to make sure you have the correct record—you must click on the correct room number within the MAR.) Click on **Return to Medication Room** after reviewing the correct MAR.

- Based on your care for Piya Jordan, access the various storage areas of the Medication Room to obtain the necessary medications you need to administer.

- For each area you access, select the medication you plan to administer and then click **Put Medication on Tray**. When finished with a storage area, click on **Close Drawer** or **Close Bin**.

- Click on **View Medication Room**.

- Click on **Preparation** and choose the correct medication to administer. Click **Prepare**.

- Click **Next** and choose the correct patient to administer this medication to. Click **Finish**.

- You can **Review Your Medications** and then **Return to Medication Room** when ready. Once you are back in Medication Room, go directly to Piya Jordan's room to administer this medication by clicking on **403** at bottom of the screen.

- After you have collected the appropriate assessment data and are ready for administration, click **Patient Care** and **Medication Administration**. Verify that the correct patient and medication(s) appear in the left-hand window. Then click the down arrow next to Select. From the drop-down menu, select **Administer** and complete the Administration Wizard by providing any information requested. When the Wizard stops asking for information, click **Administer to Patient**. Specify **Yes** when asked whether this administration should be recorded in the MAR. Finally, click **Finish**.

10. Below is a list of steps describing the proper technique for administering an IV push medication. Indicate the correct sequence by numbering the steps from 1 to 10.

_____ a. Clean off injection port with antiseptic swab.

_____ b. Recheck fluid infusion rate.

_____ c. Perform hand hygiene and apply gloves.

_____ d. Select injection port of IV tubing closest to patient.

_____ e. Check patient's identification by looking at identification bracelet and asking patient's name.

_____ f. Occlude IV line and check for blood return.

_____ g. Withdraw syringe from port.

_____ h. Connect syringe to IV line.

_____ i. Dispose of uncapped needles and syringe and perform hand hygiene.

_____ j. Release tubing and inject medication within time recommended.

11. After administering ondansetron, how would you evaluate Piya Jordan for side effects or adverse reactions to the drug?

12. Headache, chest pain, and difficulty breathing can be side effects of ondansetron. If Piya Jordan developed these, what would you do?

13. Checking a patient's identification bracelet before administering a medication ensures that you:
    a. administer the medication at the Right Time.
    b. administer the medication to the Right Patient.
    c. administer the Right Medication.
    d. administer the medication with the Right Documentation.

Exercise 3

 CD-ROM Activity

 30 minutes

 In this exercise you will visit Kathryn Doyle, a 79-year-old Caucasian female who entered the skilled nursing unit after repair of an intertrochanteric fracture 2 weeks ago. You may have worked with Kathryn Doyle previously if you already completed Lesson 4, 6, 7, or 8.

- Sign in to work at Pacific View Regional Hospital on the Skilled Nursing Floor for Period of Care 2. (*Note:* If you are already in the virtual hospital from a previous exercise, click on **Leave the Floor** and then **Restart the Program** to get to the sign-in window.)
- From the Patient List, select Kathryn Doyle (Room 503).
- Click on **Get Report**.
- Click on **Go to Nurses' Station**.
- Click on **Chart** and then on **503**.
- Click on and review the **History and Physical**.
- Click on the **Physician's Orders**.
- Next, click on and review the **Nurse's Notes**.

1. From what you know about Kathryn Doyle in the clinical report, in what way can the administration of oral medications become a useful therapy for one of her clinical problems?

2. Match each of the medications ordered for Kathryn Doyle with the appropriate medication purpose(s).

Medication	**Purpose**
_____ Calcium citrate	a. Treatment for anemia
_____ Ferrous sulfate	b. Prevention of infection
_____ Docusate sodium	c. Prevention of constipation
_____ Ibuprofen	d. Treatment for osteoporosis
	e. Improvement of appetite
	f. Relief of pain in left hip

- Click on **Return to Nurses' Station**.
- Click on **Medication Room**.

3. What should you check before beginning to remove medications from the dispensing system? (Place an X next to all that apply.)

_____ a. Patient's fluid intake for last 8 hours

_____ b. Patient's vital signs at 0700

_____ c. Patient's Medication Administration Record

_____ d. Patient's activity order

_____ e. Patient's allergy record

- Review the patient's MAR to determine the medications that Kathryn Doyle is ordered to receive. (*Note:* You may click on **Review MAR** at any time to verify correct medication order. Remember to look at the patient name on MAR to make sure you have the correct record—you must click on the correct room number within the MAR.) Click on **Return to Medication Room** after reviewing the correct MAR.
- Based on your care for Kathryn Doyle access the various storage areas of the Medication Room to obtain the necessary medications you need to administer.
- For each area you access, select the medication you plan to administer and then click **Put Medication on Tray**. When finished with a storage area, click on **Close Drawer** or **Close Bin**.
- Click on **View Medication Room**.
- Click on **Preparation** and choose the correct medication to administer. Click **Prepare**.
- Click **Next** and choose the correct patient to administer this medication to. Click **Finish**.
- You can **Review Your Medications** and then **Return to Medication Room** when ready.
- Complete questions 4 through 6 below before going to Kathryn Doyle's room to administer her medication.

4. Two of the drugs you are administering to Kathryn Doyle could cause constipation. Which drugs are they?
   a. Ferrous sulfate and docusate sodium
   b. Calcium citrate and ibuprofen
   c. Ibuprofen and ferrous sulfate
   d. Ferrous sulfate and calcium citrate

5. What is the most common side effect to be concerned with in administering ibuprofen?
   a. Gastrointestinal distress
   b. Headache
   c. Black stool
   d. Urinary frequency

6. How many times do you check the information on the MAR with the label on the medication during preparation?

→ • Click on **503** at the bottom of the screen to go to Kathryn Doyle's room.
  • Click on **Patient Care**.
  • Click on **Medication Administration**.

7. If Kathryn Doyle asked you to crush her pills and mix them with applesauce, what would be your response?

→ • After you have collected the appropriate assessment data and are ready for administration, click **Patient Care** and **Medication Administration**. Verify that the correct patient and medication(s) appear in the left-hand window. Then click the down arrow next to Select. From the drop-down menu, select **Administer** and complete the Administration Wizard by providing any information requested. When the Wizard stops asking for information, click **Administer to Patient**. Specify **Yes** when asked whether this administration should be recorded in the MAR. Finally, click **Finish**.

8. Now that you have completed administering the medications, click on **Leave the Floor** at the bottom of your screen. From the Floor Menu, select **Look at Your Preceptor's Evaluation**. Then click on **Medication Scorecard**. How did you do? Review your results.

LESSON **8** _____

Activity and Mobility

_____

/O⌒O **Reading Assignment:**   Immobility (Chapter 34)
                               Exercise and Activity (Chapter 25)

Patients: Kathryn Doyle, Skilled Nursing Floor, Room 503
                Goro Oishi, Skilled Nursing Floor, Room 505

Objectives:

- Describe the effects of immobility on body systems.
- Describe the effects of exercise on body systems.
- Perform an assessment of a patient's risk for developing complications from immobility.
- Develop a plan of care for promoting activity tolerance in a case study patient.
- Explain nursing interventions appropriate for reducing effects of immobility.
- Describe techniques for safely assisting patients with positioning and ambulation.
- Describe principles for use of assistive devices.

Patients within health care settings present a wide variety of activity and mobility limitations. As a nurse, you must be able to recognize not only how patients' presenting health problems affect their ability to remain active and mobile but also how these problems pose risks for the function of all body systems. Preventive care is a key aspect of supporting a patients' mobility and activity tolerance. Early assessment is especially important as you learn to look for changes reflecting the effects of immobilization. As a critical thinker you will learn to incorporate nursing interventions to keep patients active and to prevent complications of immobility.

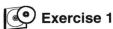 **Exercise 1**

  CD-ROM Activity

45 minutes

In this exercise you will visit Kathryn Doyle, a 79-year-old Caucasian female who was admitted following a "fall" at home in which she sustained a left hip fracture. You may have worked with Kathryn Doyle previously if you already completed Lesson 4, 6, 7, or 8.

- Sign in to work at Pacific View Regional Hospital on the Skilled Nursing Floor for Period of Care 2. (*Note:* If you are already in the virtual hospital from a previous exercise, click on **Leave the Floor** and then **Restart the Program** to get to the sign-in window.)
- From the Patient List, select Kathryn Doyle (Room 503).
- Click on **Get Report**.
- Click on **Go to Nurses' Station**.
- Click on **Chart**.
- Select the chart for Room **503**.
- Click on and review the **Nursing Admission**.
- Click on and review the **Nurse's Notes**.

1. List three bone and muscle changes that could have resulted from the immobilization of Kathryn Doyle's hip during initial treatment.

2. What is revealed in Kathryn Doyle's history that indicates her being at risk for bone fracture?

3. Using the nursing history as a data base, review the factors that are increasing Kathryn Doyle's risks for complications from immobility. Then, for each of the factors listed below, identify the systemic and psychosocial complications for which she is most at risk.

Risk Factor	Systemic/Psychosocial Complications
a. Decreased skin turgor	
b. Limited social support	
c. Concentrated dark urine	
d. Limited ROM in left lower leg and reluctance to ambulate	

4. Based on the risks noted in question 3, identify two nursing interventions you would use to minimize the effects of each potential complication.

 • Click on **Return to Nurses' Station**.
  • Click on **EPR** and then on **Login**.
  • Select **503** as the patient's room.
  • Select and review the **Nutrition** findings and then the **I&O** data.

Kathryn Doyle's history reveals a poor appetite, and she has not consistently eaten all of her meals. She is at risk for negative nitrogen balance unless she becomes more active and mobile. Fill in the blanks in the statements below.

5. Immobilization causes muscle _____, which leads to negative nitrogen balance.

6. The weight loss associated with negative nitrogen balance is due to _____ catabolism.

7. Loss of protein leads to _____ loss.

8. A person who has been immobile and develops a loss of appetite typically has a deficiency

   in calories and _____.

 • Click on **Return to Nurses' Station**.
  • Click on **Chart**.
  • Select the chart for Room **503**.
  • Click on **Consultations** and read the Physical Therapy Consult.

9. Explain why Kathryn Doyle would be given a walker instead of crutches.

10. The physical therapy note states that the left lower extremity is being given ROM. What type of ROM is this likely referring to?

11. While performing ROM exercises on the left lower leg, Kathryn Doyle complains that she is too weak to complete the exercise. What is your best option at this time?
    a. Reduce the number of exercise repetitions.
    b. Have the patient stop exercising and move the joint passively instead.
    c. Stop the exercises until the patient is willing to participate.
    d. Support the leg and foot and coach the patient to move through full ROM as much as she can.

12. When Kathryn Doyle visits physical therapy, the therapists will assist her in walking with a walker and performing ROM exercises. Complete the chart below to describe the evaluation approach for Kathryn Doyle's therapy.

Activity	Evaluation Measures	Expected Responses
Walking with walker		
ROM		

Exercise 2

CD-ROM Activity

30 minutes

In this exercise you will visit Goro Oishi, a 66-year-old Asian-American male who is admitted for hospice care following an intracerebral hemorrhage. You may have worked with Goro Oishi previously if you already completed Lesson 18.

- Sign in to work at Pacific View Regional Hospital on the Skilled Nursing Floor for Period of Care 1. (*Note:* If you are already in the virtual hospital from a previous exercise, click on **Leave the Floor** and then **Restart the Program** to get to the sign-in window.)
- From the Patient List, select Goro Oishi (Room 505).
- Click on **Get Report**.
- Click on **Go to Nurses' Station**.
- Click on **Chart**.
- Select the chart for Room **505**.
- Click on and review the **History and Physical**.
- Select **Nursing Admission** and review.

1. Goro Oishi is receiving palliative care, and thus the aim of the nurse is to manage symptoms and minimize the development of discomforting complications. What nursing measure can the nurse initiate that will reduce the patient's risk for pressure ulcer formation and improve his ability to breathe with less effort?

2. Goro Oishi is currently lying on his right side with head of bed elevated 20 degrees, and you want to turn him to his left side. Indicate the correct sequence by numbering the following steps from 1 to 13. (Step 1 has been numbered for you.)

    _____ Place pillow behind patient's back.

    _____ Have each nurse grasp drawsheet firmly near the patient.

    _____ Flex patient's right knee.

    _____ Place pillow under semiflexed right leg level at hip from groin to foot.

    _____ Remove any pillows and roll patient over to assume the supine position.

    __**1**__ Obtain assistance from another nurse and raise bed to working height.

    _____ Have nurse on left side of bed place one hand on patient's hip and one hand on shoulder; then roll client toward the left.

    _____ Lower side rails and position a nurse on each side of bed.

    _____ Place pillow under patient's head and neck and bring left shoulder blade forward.

    _____ Assuming the proper stance, coordinate with the other nurse and lift the patient to align just to the right side of bed.

    _____ Lower head of bed until it is flat.

    _____ Position both arms in slightly flexed position.

    _____ Place a sandbag parallel to plantar surface of right foot.

3. The clinical report noted that Goro Oishi has an elevated body temperature. Name two ways this can increase the risks associated with immobilization.

Oxygenation

Reading Assignment: Oxygenation (Chapter 28)

Patients: Patricia Newman, Medical-Surgical Floor, Room 406
Jacquline Catanazaro, Medical-Surgical Floor, Room 402

Objectives:

- Describe factors that can alter oxygenation.
- Explain the relationship between cardiac and respiratory alterations.
- Identify the influence that physiologic changes in oxygenation have on a patient's clinical condition.
- Identify lifestyle risk factors for problems with oxygenation.
- Apply critical thinking in the assessment of a case study patient.
- Identify nursing diagnoses that apply to a case study patient.
- Explain the rationale for use of specific nursing interventions for patients in the case studies.
- Identify the approach to evaluate patients' responses to oxygenation therapies.

The normal function of the cardiac and respiratory systems in delivering oxygen is necessary to sustain life. In the care of patients with oxygenation alterations, it is important for you as the nurse to understand cardiovascular and respiratory physiology. This knowledge base will allow you to better understand assessment data, select appropriate nursing diagnoses and plan relevant nursing interventions.

Changes in a patient's oxygenation can be the result of acute or chronic disease conditions. Patients in acute respiratory distress will be anxious and fearful, requiring your timely and attentive care. Patients with chronic respiratory disorders will require your support in understanding the long-term implications of an illness and your assistance in adapting their lifestyle.

Exercise 1

 CD-ROM Activity

 45 minutes

 Patricia Newman is a 61-year-old Caucasian female with a history of emphysema for 12 years. She has been admitted to the emergency department in moderate respiratory distress. You may have worked with Patricia Newman previously if you already completed Lesson 2, 3, 5, 9, or 10.

• Sign in to work at Pacific View Regional Hospital on the Medical-Surgical Floor for Period of Care 1. (*Note:* If you are already in the virtual hospital from a previous exercise, click on **Leave the Floor** and then **Restart the Program** to get to the sign-in window.)

• From the Patient List, select Patricia Newman (Room 406).

• Click on **Get Report** and review the clinical report summary.

• Click on **Go to Nurses' Station**.

• Click on **Chart**.

• Select the chart for Room **406**.

• Click on and review the **History and Physical**.

• Click on and review the patient's **Laboratory Reports**.

1. Patricia Newman is 61 years old. Let's assume that she has smoked since the age of 22. If so, how many packs of cigarettes would she have averaged on a daily basis? (*Study Tip:* Apply the formula for pack-year history.)

2. Patricia Newman has been diagnosed with pneumonia. Which of the following physiologic changes in oxygenation result from pneumonia? (Place an X next to all that apply.)

_____ a. Impaired ventilatory movement

_____ b. Decreased hemoglobin level

_____ c. Decreased diffusion of oxygen from the alveoli to the blood

_____ d. Inability of tissues to extract oxygen from the blood

_____ e. Obstruction of airways with mucus

3. Patricia Newman also has emphysema, a form of chronic obstructive pulmonary disease. For each of the following physiologic changes that result from emphysema, provide a rationale.

Physiologic Change	Rationale
Increased work of breathing	
Fatigue	
Dyspnea on exertion	
Elevated $PaCO_2$	

➔ • While still in the patient's chart, review the **Nursing Admission**.

4. As you review the data in Patricia Newman's H&P and Nursing Admission, apply the critical thinking model in your assessment of the patient. Complete the following critical thinking diagram for assessment of Patricia Newman's situation by writing the letter of each critical thinking factor under its proper category.

Knowledge

1. _____

2. _____

3. _____

Experience

4. _____

5. _____

ASSESSMENT OXYGENATION

Standards

8. _____

9. _____

10. _____

Attitudes

6. _____

7. _____

Critical Thinking Factors

a. Patricia Newman shows a pattern of poor health promotion practices. Explore and learn more about the patient to understand the reason for her behavior.

b. Apply what you know about respiratory physiology to determine the effects emphysema has on rate and depth of breathing.

c. The time you cared for a patient with pneumonia in the health clinic will help you recognize Patricia Newman's presenting symptoms.

d. Compare the ranges of normal laboratory values with Patricia Newman's test results.

e. Each time you auscultate lung sounds, be sure to follow the same pattern for placement of the stethoscope as you listen to all lobes of the lung.

f. Refer to nutrition therapy principles when you assess the patient's diet history.

g. If you are uncertain about how to interpret arterial blood gas levels, read a reference on acid-base balance.

h. Reflect on the time you cared for a patient with emphysema in the past. How did that patient adjust to the need to follow a medication schedule, and what is similar about Patricia Newman?

i. Refer to pharmacology sources in reviewing the effects of Patricia Newman's medications on her blood pressure.

j. When auscultating the patient's blood pressure, be sure the cuff is applied correctly to her arm and that you inflate the cuff 30 mm Hg above the point at which palpable pulse disappears.

• Click on **Return to Nurses' Station**.
 • Click on Room **406** at the bottom of the screen.
 • Review the **Initial Observations.**
 • Click on **Patient Care**.
 • Click on **Physical Assessment** and review the assessments for Head & Neck, Chest, and Back & Spine.

 5. When auscultating Patricia Newman's lung sounds, what sounds would you expect as a result of pneumonia? Give a rationale. (*Study Tip:* Review thorax and lung assessment in Chapter 13 in your textbook.)

6. Patricia Newman has sinus tachycardia as a result of which of the following factors? (Place an X next to all that apply.)

_____ a. Tobacco use

_____ b. Estrogen patch use

_____ c. Pain

_____ d. Hypoxia

_____ e. Hypertension

7. Patricia Newman's assessment reveals the following physical findings: PaCO$_2$ 47; dyspnea on exertion; naps frequently; abnormal rate and depth of breathing. Based on these findings, what is the most appropriate nursing diagnosis?

a. Ineffective breathing pattern
b. Ineffective tissue perfusion
c. Impaired gas exchange
d. Ineffective airway clearance

8. Give a rationale for the nursing diagnosis you chose in question 7.

9. For the nursing diagnosis of Impaired Gas Exchange, list two outcomes that you would develop in a plan of care to address the goal of "Patient will experience improved gas exchange."

10. What is the stimulus for Patricia Newman to breathe? What is the normal stimulus to breathe?

Exercise 2

 CD-ROM Activity

 30 minutes

 Patricia Newman is a 61-year-old Caucasian female with a history of emphysema for 12 years. She has been admitted to the emergency department in moderate respiratory distress. You may have worked with Patricia Newman previously if you completed Lesson 2, 3, 5, 9, or 10.

- Sign in to work at Pacific View Regional Hospital on the Medical-Surgical Floor for Period of Care 2. (*Note:* If you are already in the virtual hospital from a previous exercise, click on **Leave the Floor** and then **Restart the Program** to get to the sign-in window.)
- From the Patient List, select Patricia Newman (Room 406).
- Click on **Get Report** and review.
- Click on **Go to Nurses' Station**.
- Click on **Chart**.
- Select the chart for Room **406**.
- Review the **History and Physical**.

1. Complete the chart below for Patricia Newman's arterial blood gas values. (*Study Tip:* Review acid-base balance in Chapter 15 in your textbook.)

Blood Gas Value	Normal or Abnormal?	Reason for Abnormal Values
pH 7.33		
PaO$_2$ 70		
HCO$_3$ 26		
CO$_2$ 47		

2. List three lifestyle risk factors that likely contribute to Patricia Newman's emphysema and hypertension.

 • Review the **Nursing Admission**.

3. Patricia Newman's history reveals poor adherence to health promotion behaviors. As her nurse, what recommendations might you make to prevent future occurrences of pneumonia?

 • Click on **Return to the Nurses' Station**.
• Click on **406** to go to Patricia Newman's room.
• Review the **Initial Observations.**
• Select **Patient Care**.
• Click on **Nurse-Client Interactions**.
• Select and view the video titled **1100: Care Coordination**. (*Note:* If this video is not available, check the virtual clock to see whether enough time has elapsed. The video cannot be viewed before its specified time.)

4. Patricia Newman has a number of health problems. Listed below are nursing diagnoses that apply to her. Draw a concept map in the figure provided by showing the connection between the nursing diagnoses. (*Study Tip:* See pages 121-122 in your textbook.)

Impaired Gas Exchange

Fatigue

Imbalanced Nutrition: Less Than Body Requirements

Ineffective Health Maintenance

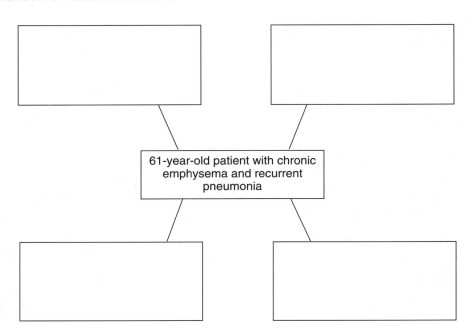

61-year-old patient with chronic emphysema and recurrent pneumonia

➤ • Click on **Return to Nurses' Station**.
  • Click on **Chart**.
  • Select the chart for Room **406**.
  • Review the **Patient Education** file.

5. Match the recommended therapy on the left with the rationale on the right.

Therapy	Rationale
_____ Use of metered-dose inhaler	a. Promotes airway clearance
_____ Perform pursed-lip breathing	b. Reduces degree of dyspnea
_____ Increase periods of walking to 20 minutes 2 times a day	c. Dilates airways reducing airflow resistance
_____ Perform effective cascade cough	d. Maintains normal mucociliary clearance
_____ Increase fluids to 3 liters per day	e. Prevents alveolar collapse

6. In addition to pursed-lip breathing, what other breathing exercise might you teach Patricia Newman? Explain.

Patricia Newman is receiving oxygen 2 liters per minute by nasal cannula. Select true or false for questions 7 through 11.

7. Increasing the flow rate on a nasal cannula oxygen device to 6 liters per minute will significantly increase delivered oxygen concentration.
   a. True
   b. False

8. A flow rate of 2 liters per minute delivers approximately 24%-28% oxygen
   a. True
   b. False

9. An oxygen mask is a delivery device that would be contraindicated for Patricia Newman.
   a. True
   b. False

10. When placing patients on oxygen, attach a humidified oxygen source to reduce nasal mucosal drying.
    a. True
    b. False

11. Because Patricia Newman's PaO$_2$ is 70, she might benefit from receiving oxygen by a Venturi mask.
    a. True
    b. False

Exercise 3

 CD-ROM Activity

 30 minutes

 Jacquline Catanazaro is a 45-year-old female with a 30-year history of asthma, complicated by schizophrenia. She has been admitted to the ED because of an acute asthma episode and concurrent schizophrenic episode. You may have worked with Jacquline Catanazaro previously if you completed Lesson 13.

• Sign in to work at Pacific View Regional Hospital on the Medical-Surgical Floor for Period of Care 1. (*Note:* If you are already in the virtual hospital from a previous exercise, click on **Leave the Floor** and then **Restart the Program** to get to the sign-in window.)

• From the Patient List, select Jacquline Catanazaro (Room 402).

• Click on **Get Report**.

• Click on **Go to Nurses' Station**.

• Click on **Chart**.

• Select the chart for Room **402**.

• Click on and review the **Nursing Admission**.

1. Explain how Jacquline Catanazaro's obesity affects her ability to breathe.

2. Jacquline Catanazaro reportedly can become very anxious from her mental illness. Which of the following best describes the influence anxiety has on the patient's oxygenation status?
   a. Causes hypoventilation
   b. Increases the body's metabolic rate and oxygen demand
   c. Reduces the diffusion of oxygen across the alveolar membrane
   d. Creates a sense of breathlessness from CO_2 retention

3. The physician ordered stat nebulization for Jacquline Catanazaro using albuterol. Nebulization will most likely improve her ability to breathe by what mechanism? (*Study Tip:* Refer to your pharmacology text for albuterol's action.)

   _____ a. Decreasing the volume of sputum to expectorate

   _____ b. Cooling inhaled air

   _____ c. Relieving bronchospasm

   _____ d. Enhancing mucociliary clearance

   _____ e. Reducing the patient's peak flow rate

→ • Click on **Go to Nurses' Station**.
   • Select Room **402** at the bottom of the screen.
   • Review the **Initial Observations.**
   • Select **Patient Care** and then click on **Nurse-Client Interactions**.
   • Select and view the video titled **0730: Intervention—Airway**. (*Note:* If this video is not available, check the virtual clock to see whether enough time has elapsed. The video cannot be viewed before its specified time.)
   • Next, click on **Physical Assessment** and conduct a focused assessment based on Jacquline Catanazaro's current condition.

4. Match Jacquline Catanazaro's physical findings on the left with the physiologic change on the right.

Physical Findings	Physiologic Change
_____ Hyperresonance to percussion	a. Increased airway resistance
_____ Substernal retraction	b. High-velocity airflow
_____ Tachypnea	c. Air-filled lungs
_____ Wheezes bilaterally	d. Decreased oxygen levels trigger increased respiratory rate
_____ Peak flow meter shows value of 200	e. Increased work of breathing

• Click on **Return to Nurses' Station**.
- Click on **Leave the Floor**.
- From the Floor Menu, select **Restart the Program**.
- Sign in to care for Jacquline Catanazaro on the Medical-Surgical Floor for Period of Care 2.
- Click on **Go to Nurses' Station**.
- Click on **Chart**.
- Select the chart for Room **402**.
- Select the **Physician's Notes** and review.
- Select the **Physician's Orders** and review.

5. The physician's notes for 0800 and 1000 show two sets of arterial blood gases:

   0800: pH 7.38, PaO_2 80, $PaCO_2$ 50, HCO_3 26, Oxygen saturation 85%

   1000: pH 7.40, PaO_2 92, $PaCO_2$ 40, HCO_3 23, Oxygen saturation 99%

   a. Explain the reason for the change in this patient's blood gases.

   b. Are Jacquline Catazanaro's ABGs now normal?

6. Considering that Jacquline Catanazaro has a productive cough with frothy secretions, why would it be inadvisable to perform tracheal suctioning?

10

Managing Fluid and Electrolyte Balance

/OℛƆ **Reading Assignment:**   Fluids, Electrolytes, and Acid-Base Balances (Chapter 15)
Oxygenation (Chapter 28)
Care of Surgical Clients (Chapter 37)

Patients: Piya Jordan, Medical-Surgical Floor, Room 403
Patricia Newman, Medical-Surgical Floor, Room 406

Objectives:

- Identify disturbances in fluids and electrolytes in case study patients.
- Identify acid-base imbalances in case study patients.
- Explain the function of electrolytes.
- Apply critical thinking in the assessment of a patient for fluid and electrolyte imbalance.
- Describe variables that affect fluid and electrolyte balance.
- Describe factors to include in the assessment of a peripheral intravenous site.
- Calculate an intravenous flow rate.
- Describe the risks associated with blood transfusion.
- Identify steps used in the insertion of a peripheral intravenous catheter.

Fluid, electrolyte, and acid-base balances within the body are needed to maintain the health and function of all body systems. As a nurse it is important to understand what physiologic changes occur from fluid and electrolyte and acid-base imbalances, the risks a patient has for imbalance, and the types of therapies used to reverse imbalance. An important responsibility is to monitor patients closely for fluid and electrolyte or acid-base changes. A patient's condition can change very quickly, thus requiring a nurse's astute observation and timely action.

Competency in the safe and effective administration of intravenous fluid therapy is critical to management of fluid and electrolyte and acid-base alterations. This includes knowing how to correctly establish IV access, monitoring and calculating IV infusions, and maintaining infusion systems. How well you manage IV infusion therapy may determine your patient's clinical course.

Exercise 1

  CD-ROM Activity

 45 minutes

In this exercise you will visit Piya Jordan, a 68-year-old Asian-American female who entered the hospital after an emergency department admission for abdominal pain, nausea, and vomiting. She underwent abdominal surgery for the removal of a mass in her right lower quadrant. You may have worked with Piya Jordan previously if you already completed Lesson 7 or 15.

- Sign in to work at Pacific View Regional Hospital on the Medical-Surgical Floor for Period of Care 1. (*Note:* If you are already in the virtual hospital from a previous exercise, click on **Leave the Floor** and then **Restart the Program** to get to the sign-in window.)
- From the Patient List, select Piya Jordan (Room 403).
- Click on **Get Report**.
- Click on **Go to Nurses' Station**.
- Click on **Chart**.
- Click on the chart for Room **403**.
- Review the **Nursing Admission**.

1. Identify three factors in Piya Jordan's Nursing Admission data that explain her risks for fluid and electrolyte imbalance prior to surgery.

2. Consider the data you received from the clinical report summary. From the following list, identify the risks Piya Jordan has for fluid and electrolyte imbalance postoperatively.

_____ a. Taking digoxin at home

_____ b. Nasogastric tube draining moderate brown fluid

_____ c. Intravenous infusion of D_5 NS with 20 mEq KCl

_____ d. Receiving meperidine via patient controlled analgesia

_____ e. Patient is NPO

_____ f. Telemetry shows atrial fibrillation

➤ • Still in the chart, click on **Laboratory Reports** and review the chemistry findings.

3. Complete the chart below by listing Piya Jordan's chemistry results. Note whether values show a normal or abnormal trend.

Lab Value	Mon 2200	Tues 0630	Wed 0630	Result Normal/Abnormal
Na				
K				
Cl				
CO_2				
BUN				

4. As a result of Piya Jordan's trend toward hypokalemia, which of the following signs and symptoms would she most likely experience? (Place an X next to all that apply.)

_____ a. Confusion

_____ b. Abnormal ventricular arrhythmias

_____ c. Flushed skin

_____ d. Weakness and fatigue

_____ e. Thirst

_____ f. Decreased bowel sounds

_____ g. Diarrhea

➤ • Click on and review the **History and Physical**.

5. Piya Jordan's BUN is elevated. The BUN is a measure of urea in the blood and is an indication of the excretory function of the kidney. Why might the BUN be elevated preoperatively? What treatment did she receive to help reverse this?

6. Piya Jordan's postoperative care will require you as the nurse to conduct a thorough assessment. Critical thinking applied to assessment enables you to develop a relevant plan of care. Complete the following critical thinking diagram for assessment of Piya Jordan's situation by writing the letter of each critical thinking factor under its proper category.

Knowledge

1. _____

2. _____

3. _____

Experience   **PLANNING**   **Standards**

4. _____   5. _____

6. _____

7. _____

Attitudes

8. _____

Critical Thinking Factors

a. Be very thorough in your approach to assessment, take time to examine the abdominal wound and dressing, and do not rush yourself.
b. When measuring Piya Jordan's output from the JP tube, use a measured container.
c. Review the physiology of the effect surgery has on fluid and electrolyte balance.
d. Consider how a surgical alteration of the colon will affect fluid and electrolyte balance.
e. As you assess Piya Jordan, consider the appearance of the skin and mucous membranes in previous patients you have cared for.
f. Refer to the Infusion Nurse's Society infiltration and phlebitis scales when examining Piya Jordan's IV site.
g. Be aware of normal physical assessment findings as you compare findings from your examination of Piya Jordan.
h. Consider what you know about signs and symptoms of electrolyte alterations.

• Click on **Return to Nurses' Station**.
• Click on Room **403** at the bottom of the screen.
• Review the **Initial Observations.**

7. Piya Jordan's IV is running at 100 mL/hr. Assuming the IV is being delivered via a macro-drip tubing, compute the drop rates for each of the two different drop factors below.

Drop factor	Drop rate (gtt/mL)
IV drop factor 10gtt/mL	
IV drop factor 15 gtt/mL	

- Click on **Patient Care**.
- Click on **Physical Assessment**.
- Review the assessment categories that you believe pertain to Piya Jordan's fluid and electrolyte status.

8. During Piya Jordan's Head & Neck assessment, the subcategories of Gastrointestinal and Integumentary reveal the following: oral mucosa pink and moist, skin warm and moist. What do these findings indicate?

9. Observe the photo of Piya Jordan's IV site during the Upper Extremities assessment. What is wrong with the dressing?

10. Which of the following best describes an IV site without complications?
    a. IV infusing at 75 mL/hr, site warm with redness, nontender
    b. IV infusing at 100 mL/hr, site nontender, without redness or swelling
    c. IV infusing at keep-vein-open rate, swelling less than 1 inch around site, cool to touch
    d. IV infusing at 100 mL/hr, pain on palpation over site, skin blanched and cool to touch

- Click on **Return to Nurses' Station**.
- Click on the **EPR**.
- Click on **Login**.
- Choose **403** from the Patient drop-down menu; select **I&O** as the category.
- Review the I&O for Piya Jordan between 2300 on Tuesday and 0700 Wednesday.

11. What was Piya Jordan's fluid balance (intake minus output) for the 8-hour period 2300 to 0700?

12. Which of the following interventions would be appropriate in Piya Jordan's case to manage the fluid imbalance?
    a. Give the patient oral liquids
    b. Increase the infusion rate of the IV
    c. Give the patient tube feeding
    d. Discontinue NG decompression

Exercise 2

 CD-ROM Activity

 45 minutes

 In this exercise you will visit Piya Jordan, a 68-year-old Asian-American female who entered the hospital after an emergency department admission for abdominal pain, nausea, and vomiting. She underwent abdominal surgery for the removal of a mass in her right lower quadrant. You may have worked with Piya Jordan previously if you already completed Lesson 7 or 15.

• Sign in to work at Pacific View Regional Hospital on the Medical-Surgical Floor for Period of Care 2. (*Note:* If you are already in the virtual hospital from a previous exercise, click on **Leave the Floor** and then **Restart the Program** to get to the sign-in window.)
• From the Patient List, select Piya Jordan (Room 403).
• Click on **Get Report**.
• Click on **Go to Nurses' Station**.
• Click on **Chart**.
• Click on the chart for Room **403**.
• Click on the **History and Physical**.
• Review the **Physician's Orders**.
• Next, click on and review the **Laboratory Reports**.

1. The surgeon has ordered 2 units of packed red blood cells to be administered to Piya Jordan for a low hemoglobin and hematocrit. What caused the drop in her hemoglobin and hematocrit?

2. The laboratory reports indicate that Piya Jordan's blood type is A+. Complete the chart below by filling in each box as it applies to Piya Jordan.

Patient's Blood Type	Red Blood Cell Antigen	Transfuse with Type A?	Transfuse with Type B?	Transfuse with Type AB?	Transfuse with Type O?

3. What does the positive (+) indicate for Piya Jordan's blood type?

➤ • Click on the **Nurse's Notes**.

4. The nurse's notes indicate that the nurse "explained precautions" related to blood procurement. Which of the following is the correct procedure to ensure a patient receives the right blood product?
   a. When checking the blood label, have the nurse administering the blood check the patient's name.
   b. When checking the blood label, have two designated staff check the label for the blood type.
   c. When checking the blood label, have two designated staff check it against the patient's name, identification number, and the blood type.
   d. When checking the label, have the nurse administering the blood ask the patient to identify his or her blood type.

5. The physician orders a saline lock to be inserted for the administration of 2 units of packed cells. Show the correct sequence of steps for inserting a saline lock by numbering the steps below from 1 to 13.

   _____ a. Release tourniquet temporarily.

   _____ b. Look for blood return and advance catheter into vein; loosen and remove stylet.

   _____ c. Prepare an IV bag, tubing, and saline lock, filling tubing and lock with normal saline.

   _____ d. Select a vein large enough for catheter placement. Palpate vein and promote venous distention.

   _____ e. Perform hand hygiene.

   _____ f. Perform venipuncture. Puncture skin and vein, holding catheter at 10- to 30-degree angle. Insert with bevel up.

   _____ g. Stabilize the catheter, apply pressure above insertion site, and release tourniquet.

   _____ h. Apply disposable gloves.

   _____ i. Reapply tourniquet.

   _____ j. Identify an accessible vein; apply tourniquet.

   _____ k. Cleanse insertion site.

   _____ l. Connect adapter from fluid infusion tubing and saline lock to catheter hub.

   _____ m. Release roller clamp and regulate infusion rate.

Fill in the blanks in the following questions.

6. Before a transfusion begins, the nurse obtains a patient's baseline _____ signs.

7. The initiation of a transfusion begins _____ to allow for early detection of a transfusion reaction.

8. The nurse stays with a patient during the first _____ minutes, the time when a transfusion reaction is most likely to occur.

9. A unit of packed RBCs should be transfused in _____ hours.

10. If the patient develops chills, fever, tachycardia, and tachypnea, the first action is to

_____ the transfusion.

Exercise 3

CD-ROM Activity

30 minutes

Patricia Newman is a 61-year-old Caucasian female with a history of emphysema for 12 years. She has been admitted to the emergency department in moderate respiratory distress. You may have worked with Patricia Newman previously if you completed Lesson 2, 3, 5, 9, or 10.

- Sign in to work at Pacific View Regional Hospital on the Medical-Surgical Floor for Period of Care 1. (*Note:* If you are already in the virtual hospital from a previous exercise, click on **Leave the Floor** and then **Restart the Program** to get to the sign-in window.)
- From the Patient List, select Patricia Newman (Room 406).
- Click on **Get Report**.
- Click on **Go to Nurses' Station**.
- Click on **Chart**.
- Click on the chart for Room **406**.
- Review the **Nursing Admission**.

1. The clinical report summary reveals the following blood gas findings: pH 7.33, O_2 70, HCO_3 26, CO_2 47, O_2 sat 92%

   a. Answer the questions below to help you determine what type of acid-base imbalance this indicates.

   Acidosis or alkalosis? pH =

   Patient's primary physical alteration is metabolic or respiratory?

   If source of imbalance is metabolic, expect:

   If source of imbalance is respiratory, expect:

   b. The type of imbalance is:

• Click on the **History and Physical**.

 2. What condition has originally caused Patricia Newman to have this alteration in blood gases? (*Study Tip:* Review pages 774-778 in your textbook.)
   a. Hypertension
   b. Emphysema
   c. Low flow of oxygen via cannula
   d. Pneumonia

3. Alteration in respiratory function can be caused by three different primary alterations. Which of these apply to the emphysema affecting Patricia Newman?
   a. Hypoventilation
   b. Hyperventilation
   c. Hypoxia

4. Patricia Newman's pneumonia complicates her respiratory condition by causing which of the following?
   a. Hypoventilation
   b. Hyperventilation
   c. Hypoxia

 5. What physiologic stimulus causes Patricia Newman to breathe? (*Study Tip:* Review Chapter 28 in your textbook.)

 • Click on **Return to Nurses' Station**.
   • Click on **406** to go to Patricia Newman's room.
   • Review the **Initial Observations.**
   • Click on **Patient Care**.
   • Select and review the physical assessments of the **Chest & Back** and the **Spine**.

6. Place an X next to the symptom most likely to be the result of respiratory acidosis.

   _____ a. Mild dyspnea

   _____ b. Normal heart sounds

   _____ c. Sinus tachycardia

   _____ d. Coarse crackles

 • Click on **Chart**.
   • Select the chart for Room **406**.
   • Review the **Physician's Orders**.
   • Review the **Patient Education** notes.

7. To better manage the patient's acid-base imbalance, the nurse will attempt to improve Patricia Newman's oxygenation. Match the nursing interventions on the left with the rationales on the right.

Nursing Intervention	**Rationale**
_____ Encourage effective coughing	a. Opens bronchioles to enhance oxygen and carbon dioxide exchange
_____ Instruct patient to perform pursed-lip breathing	b. Relieves hypoxia and helps to minimize dyspnea
_____ Administer bronchodilator by metered-dose inhaler	c. Removes secretions that alter diffusion of O_2 and CO_2
_____ Promote fluid intake	d. Reduces thick tenacious secretions that hinder gas diffusion
_____ Administer O_2 at 2 liters per nasal cannula	e. Prevents alveolar collapse and thus improves O_2 diffusion

LESSON 11

Sleep

 Reading Assignment: Sleep (Chapter 29)

Patients: Pablo Rodriguez, Medical-Surgical Floor, Room 404
William Jefferson, Skilled Nursing Floor, Room 501

Objectives:

- Identify factors that disrupt sleep in case study patients.
- Describe the relationship between disturbed sleep pattern and other nursing diagnoses.
- Develop a plan of care to promote sleep for a case study patient.
- Describe interventions designed to promote sleep.
- Identify approaches used to evaluate a patient's sleep status.

Proper rest and sleep are essential to good health. As a nurse you will care for patients who often have preexisting sleep disturbances or who develop sleep problems as a result of illness or the experience of hospitalization. To best assist patients, you must understand the nature of sleep, the factors influencing it, and a patient's sleep habits. Each patient is unique in regard to his or her sleep pattern. Patients require an individualized approach based on personal habits and pattern of sleep, as well as the particular problems influencing sleep. Your intervention can be effective in resolving both short-term and long-term sleep problems.

Exercise 1

 CD-ROM Activity

 45 minutes

In this exercise you will visit Pablo Rodriguez, a 71-year-old Hispanic male who is suffering from advanced non-small-cell lung carcinoma. You may have worked with Pablo Rodriguez previously if you already completed Lesson 6, 12, 13, or 19.

- Sign in to work at Pacific View Regional Hospital on the Medical-Surgical Floor for Period of Care 1. (*Note:* If you are already in the virtual hospital from a previous exercise, click on **Leave the Floor** and then **Restart the Program** to get to the sign-in window.)
- From the Patient List, select Pablo Rodriguez (Room 405).
- Click on **Get Report**.
- Click on **Go to Nurses' Station**.

137

- Click on **Chart**.
- Select the chart for Room **405**.
- Click on the **Nursing Admission**.

1. Place an X next to each of the factors in Pablo Rodriguez's history that are contributing to his sleep problem.

   _____ a. Eats spicy cheese and refried beans

   _____ b. Smoked 60 pack years

   _____ c. Depression

   _____ d. Takes celecoxib at home

   _____ e. Pain from subcutaneous nodules

   _____ f. Dyspnea when lying flat

2. Pablo Rodriguez reports "poor sleep and restlessness" when admitted to the hospital. His Nursing Admission notes that he sleeps 6 to 8 hours and then naps 1 to 2 times a day. List three questions to ask to better clarify his sleep pattern.

- Click on **Return to Nurses' Station**.
- Click on Room **405** at the bottom of the screen.
- Click on **Patient Care**.
- Click on **Nurse-Client Interactions**.
- Select and view the video titled **0730: Symptom Management**. (*Note:* If this video is not available, check the virtual clock to see whether enough time has elapsed. The video cannot be viewed before its specified time.)

True or False. Pablo Rodriguez is obviously experiencing emotional distress as a result of his illness. Information from his Nursing Admission further confirms this. Select true or false for questions 3 through 5.

3. Emotional stress may cause a person to try too hard to fall asleep.
   a. True
   b. False

4. Older adults who experience depressive moods often have later appearance of REM sleep.
   a. True
   b. False

5. Depression can cause a person to have frequent and early awakening.
   a. True
   b. False

6. Listed below are signs and symptoms revealed in Pablo Rodriguez's Nursing Admission and initial clinical summary. Group the signs and symptoms into four clusters reflecting four different health problems. To form the four clusters, number each of the signs or symptoms with a 1, 2, 3, or 4 to indicate which group it belongs to.

Signs and Symptoms

_____   a. Breathing labored

_____   b. Verbal complaint of not feeling rested

_____   c. Aversion to food from smell of food

_____   d. Pain reported 8 on scale of 0 to 10

_____   e. Trouble falling asleep

_____   f. Nausea

_____   g. Dyspnea when lying flat

_____   h. Nodules painful to palpation

_____   i. Awakens after falling asleep

_____   j. Facial mask with expression of discomfort

_____   k. Tachypneic

7. Now that you have clustered the signs and symptoms (or defining characteristics), which of the following nursing diagnoses are most appropriate for Pablo Rodriguez?
   a. Fatigue; Pain; Imbalanced Nutrition: Less Than Body Requirements; Sleep Disturbance
   b. Pain; Sleep Disturbance; Anxiety; Nausea
   c. Impaired Gas Exchange; Fatigue; Nausea; Anxiety
   d. Impaired Gas Exchange; Pain; Nausea; Sleep Disturbance

8. Given Pablo Rodriguez's numerous physical problems, develop a concept map by drawing arrows to show the association between nursing diagnoses. (*Study Tip:* See pages 121-122 in your textbook.)

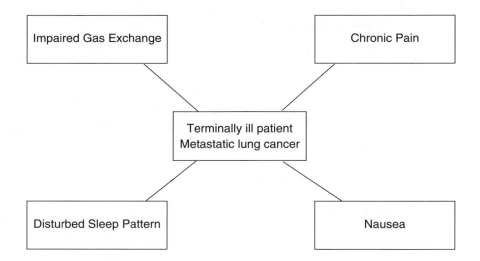

• While you are still in Pablo Rodriguez's room, select and view the video titled **0735: Patient Perceptions**. (*Note:* If this video is not available, check the virtual clock to see whether enough time has elapsed. The video cannot be viewed before its specified time.)

9. For the nursing diagnosis of Disturbed Sleep Pattern, identify four possible related factors.

10. Pablo Rodriguez's sleep problem is best described as:
    a. sleep apnea.
    b. insomnia.
    c. sleep deprivation.
    d. excessive daytime sleepiness.

11. Develop a nursing plan of care for this nursing diagnosis: Disturbed Sleep Pattern related to pain, nausea, depression, and dyspnea. In the care plan below, fill in additional goals, outcomes, interventions, and rationales. (*Study Tip:* You may have to refer to Chapters 28 and 31 in your textbook for interventions and rationales.)

Nursing Diagnosis:
Disturbed Sleep Pattern related to pain, nausea, depression, and dyspnea

Goals

1. Patient will achieve an improved sense of sleep

2.

Outcomes

1.

2. Patient will report being able to sleep 6 hours in hospital

3.

Interventions

1. Keep HOB elevated, turn patient in position of comfort

2.

3.

4. Use culturally appropriate approach in helping patient to discuss concerns over family upon his death

Rationales

1.

2. Relief of pain and nausea eliminate physiologic distractions that cause wakefulness

3. Relieves nausea

4.

---

12. After instituting your plan of care, what three evaluation measures might you use to determine whether Pablo Rodriguez's sleep disturbance has been resolved?

Exercise 2

 CD-ROM Activity

 45 minutes

 In this exercise you will visit William Jefferson, a 75-year-old African-American male who has a history of Alzheimer's disease and various other chronic ailments. He has been admitted to the skilled nursing unit with a urinary tract infection and possible sepsis. You may have worked with William Jefferson previously if you already completed Lesson 19.

- Sign in to work at Pacific View Regional Hospital on the Skilled Nursing Floor for Period of Care 1. (*Note:* If you are already in the virtual hospital from a previous exercise, click on **Leave the Floor** and then **Restart the Program** to get to the sign-in window.)
- From the Patient List, select William Jefferson (Room 501); then click on **Get Report**.
- Click on **Go to Nurses' Station** and then on **Chart**.
- Select the chart for Room **501** and click on **Nursing Admission**.

1. William Jefferson is reported by his wife to have some difficulty with sleeping at home. What food preferences, if eaten in the evening, might be altering his ability to fall asleep? List three.

2. Mrs. Jefferson reports that she does not let her husband nap for more than 1 hour. What would be your response to this information?

→ • Click on and review the **Physician's Orders**.

3. Place an X next to those medications that may contribute to William Jefferson's sleep problem. (*Study Tip:* Refer to your pharmacology text for a complete list of medications that affect sleep.)

_____ a. Rivastigmine tartrate

_____ b. Ibuprofen

_____ c. Hydrochlorothiazide

_____ d. Enalapril maleate

_____ e. Ciprofloxacin

_____ f. Metformin

_____ g. Atenolol

4. Explain the rationale for hydrochlorothiazide affecting a patient's sleep. Does William Jefferson's history confirm such a problem?

5. Knowing the effects of the medications on William Jefferson's sleep, what action might you take?

True or False. Select true or false for questions 6 through 9.

6. Low noises within the extended-care facility, such as staff talking outside of a room, are more likely to arouse a person from stage 3 sleep.
   a. True
   b. False

7. A room that is too hot can cause a person to be restless and unable to fall asleep.
   a. True
   b. False

8. It may take up to 2 weeks before elimination of a food from the diet can restore sleep.
   a. True
   b. False

9. The herbal product Kava can cause insomnia.
   a. True
   b. False

10. Match each sleep intervention on the left with its rationale on the right.

Interventions	**Rationales**
_____ Have Mrs. Jefferson offer chamomile tea to her husband in the evening.	a. Promotes maximal ventilation
_____ Recommend that William Jefferson wear loose-fitting nightwear to bed.	b. Maintains a state of fatigue and promotes relaxation
_____ Recommend a low-running fan in the bedroom at night.	c. Prevents discomfort of full bladder
_____ Encourage the patient and his wife to take their dog for a walk 2 hours before bedtime.	d. Promotes comfort
_____ Always have William Jefferson void before going to bed.	e. Provides a mild sedative effect

LESSON 12

Comfort

👓 **Reading Assignment:** Promoting Comfort (Chapter 30)

Patients: Pablo Rodriguez, Medical-Surgical Floor, Room 405
                 Piya Jordan, Medical-Surgical Floor, Room 403

Objectives:

- Differentiate acute and chronic pain.
- Describe factors that influence pain.
- Identify presenting signs and symptoms of a patient in pain.
- Describe cultural implications in pain management.
- Apply critical thinking in the assessment of a patient in pain.
- Select appropriate pain relief interventions for patients in the case studies.
- Provide rationales for pain interventions as they apply to physiology of pain.
- Discuss principles for use of patient-controlled analgesia.
- Discuss implications for use of analgesics.
- Identify approaches for evaluating a patient's response to pain therapies.

Pain is the most common reason why individuals seek health care. The experience of pain can affect an individual physically, psychologically, socially, and economically. Because pain is a subjective experience, it becomes critical for nurses to recognize that no painful event or experience is the same. A patient's personal experiences, values, and cultural background all influence the pain experience. You must respect a patient's perception and expression of pain and partner with the patient to find the most effective pain-relief strategies.

Comfort is a concept central to the art of nursing. Through comfort nurses provide strength, hope, and assistance to patients. You must learn to combine pharmacological and nonpharmacologic pain therapies to find the most effective approach to pain control. You are ethically and legally responsible for managing pain and relieving suffering. Effective pain management reduces physical discomfort and also improves a patient's quality of life.

Exercise 1

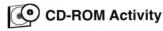 **CD-ROM Activity**

 45 minutes

 In this exercise you will visit Pablo Rodriguez, a 71-year-old Hispanic male who is suffering from advanced non-small-cell lung carcinoma. You may have worked with Pablo Rodriguez previously if you already completed Lesson 6, 11, 13, or 19.

- Sign in to work at Pacific View Regional Hospital on the Medical-Surgical Floor for Period of Care 1. (*Note:* If you are already in the virtual hospital from a previous exercise, click on **Leave the Floor** and then **Restart the Program** to get to the sign-in window.)
- From the Patient List, select Pablo Rodriguez (Room 405).
- Click on **Get Report**.
- Click on **Go to Nurses' Station**.
- Click on **Chart**.
- Select the chart for Room **405**.
- Click on and review the **Nursing Admission**.
- Click on and review the **History and Physical**.

1. Based on data from the Nursing Admission summary, list six different sources of discomfort that Pablo Rodriguez is experiencing.

2. Which of the following best describes the pain of the subcutaneous nodules?
   a. Neuropathic pain
   b. Acute pain
   c. Idiopathic pain
   d. Nociceptive somatic pain

Pablo Rodriguez is experiencing chronic pain. Select true or false for question 3 through 6.

3. Chronic pain from cancer may be sensed at the actual site of the tumor or distant to the site.
   a. True
   b. False

4. Chronic pain commonly causes fatigue, anorexia, weight loss, and insomnia.
   a. True
   b. False

5. Chronic pain usually has a predictable ending.
   a. True
   b. False

6. A common problem in the management of chronic pain is undertreatment.
   a. True
   b. False

• Click on **Return to Nurses' Station** and then on Room **405** at the bottom of the screen.
 • Review the **Initial Observations.**
 • Click on **Patient Care** and then on **Nurse-Client Interactions**.
 • Select and view the video titled **0730: Symptom Management**. (*Note:* If this video is not available, check the virtual clock to see whether enough time has elapsed. The video cannot be viewed before its specified time.)

7. Name two factors, identified within Pablo Rodriguez's admission data, that would increase his perception of pain.

8. Pablo Rodriguez's Hispanic culture influences how he experiences pain and how he is able to express it with family and caregivers. In the nursing history, the patient reported that he wishes the pain to "go away." Based on your observation of the patient during the video, which of the following statements accurately describe factors the nurse should consider in his care? (Place an X next to all that apply.)

_____ a. The nurse may need to use probing questions to thoroughly assess Pablo Rodriguez's pain.

_____ b. The patient's feelings about the meaning of pain will affect his perception of it.

_____ c. Knowing the nature of cancer pain, the nurse should presume how Pablo Rodriguez will respond.

_____ d. Whether Pablo Rodriguez is stoic or expressive about pain reflects his Hispanic culture.

_____ e. Pablo Rodriguez's language barrier makes it difficult to assess his pain.

 • Click on **EPR** at the top of your screen; then click on **Login**.
 • Specify **405** as the patient's room and **Vital Signs** as the category.
 • Review the pain assessment for Pablo Rodriguez.

9. Review the EPR findings that describe Pablo Rodriguez's pain. Place an X next to the characteristics of pain that are included in the EPR assessment.

_____ a. Pain location

_____ b. Pain intensity

_____ c. Pain onset

_____ d. Pain quality

_____ e. Behavioral effects

_____ f. Contributing factors

_____ g. Influence on activities of daily living

→ • Click on **Exit EPR** and then on **Return to Room 405.**
 • Click on **Chart**.
 • Select the chart for Room **405**.
 • Click on **Physician's Orders**.
 • Review the orders for Tuesday at 2300.

10. The EPR data indicated that relieving factors could be referred to in the MD orders. What is wrong with such an assessment finding?

11. The physician has ordered patient-controlled analgesia (PCA) with the following order: Morphine sulfate 0.5 mg IV every 10 min/12 mg in 4-hour lockout. Over a period of 1 hour, what would Pablo Rodriguez's maximal dose be?
 a. 10 mg
 b. 3 mg
 c. 30 mg
 d. 12 mg

12. If, in describing use of the PCA, Pablo Rodriguez said to you, "I am afraid to keep pushing this button so often," what would you say?

13. Morphine is an opiate. What complications does it cause that could worsen Pablo Rodriguez's current condition?

→ • Click on **Return to Nurses' Station**.
 • Click on **Leave the Floor**.
 • Click on **Restart the Program**.
 • Sign in to work at Pacific View Regional Hospital on the Medical-Surgical Floor for Period of Care 2.
 • From the Patient List, select Pablo Rodriguez (Room 405).
 • Click on **Get Report**.
 • Click on **Go to Nurses' Station**.
 • Click on **EPR**.
 • Click on **Login**.
 • Specify **405** as the patient's room.
 • Review the **Vital Signs** record for Pablo Rodriguez.

14. What does the pattern of pain severity scores tell you about Pablo Rodriguez's pain control? What intervention would you recommend after seeing this pattern of data?

15. In comparing patient-controlled analgesia with continuous IV analgesic infusions, what is the advantage of continuous IV infusion?
    a. The patient gains control over pain by accessing medication when needed.
    b. Provides a local anesthetic, avoiding systemic effects of analgesia.
    c. Avoids the serious sedative effects of parenteral narcotics.
    d. Offers uniform pain control with fewer peaks and valleys in plasma analgesic concentration.

16. Record Pablo Rodriguez's pain intensity scores for the times specified in the chart below.

	Wed 0700	Wed 0730	Wed 0900	Wed 1000	Wed 1100
Pain Score					

17. What does the pattern of pain severity scores tell you about Pablo Rodriguez's pain control? What intervention would you recommend after seeing this pattern of data?

Exercise 2

 CD-ROM Activity

 30 minutes

 In this exercise you will visit Pablo Rodriguez, a 71-year-old Hispanic male who is suffering from advanced non-small-cell lung carcinoma. You may have worked with Pablo Rodriguez previously if you already completed Lesson 6, 11, 13, or 19.

- Sign in to work at Pacific View Regional Hospital on the Medical-Surgical Floor for Period of Care 2. (*Note:* If you are already in the virtual hospital from a previous exercise, click on **Leave the Floor** and then **Restart the Program** to get to the sign-in window.)
- From the Patient List, select Pablo Rodriguez (Room 405).
- Click on **Get Report** and then on **Go to Nurses' Station**.
- Click on **Chart** and then select the chart for Room 405.
- Click on and review the **Nursing Admission**.

1. Complete the following assessment form as you review Pablo Rodriguez's clinical summary and admission data.

Age:

Activity/Rest

    Energy level:

    Sleep quality:

    Ability to perform ADLs:

    Mobility limitations:

Nutrition

    Appetite: Weight change:

    Oral cavity abnormalities:

    Nausea/vomiting?

Comfort

    Pain severity: Location:

    Quality:

    Alleviating factors:

    Aggravating factors:

Self-Concept:

2. Pablo Rodriguez's data reveal a number of nursing diagnoses. Match the defining characteristics below with four of the nursing diagnoses that apply to the patient. A defining characteristic may apply to more than one nursing diagnosis. (*Study Tip:* Refer to the NANDA international nursing diagnoses and defining characteristics listings.)

Nursing Diagnoses	**Defining Characteristics**
_____ Nausea	a. Experiencing metallic taste
_____ Chronic Pain	b. Pain reported as 5 on a scale of 0 to 10
_____ Fatigue	c. Reports difficulty falling asleep
_____ Imbalanced Nutrition: Less Than Body Requirements	d. Inability to maintain usual routines
	e. Lost 50 pounds last year
	f. Reports feeling nauseated
	g. Reports feeling weak and tired
	h. Sore, inflamed gums
	i. Loss of appetite
	j. "I am a burden"; feels guilt in not meeting responsibilities

 3. Given Pablo Rodriguez's numerous physical problems, develop a concept map by drawing arrows to show the association between nursing diagnoses. (*Study Tip:* See pages 121-122 in your textbook.)

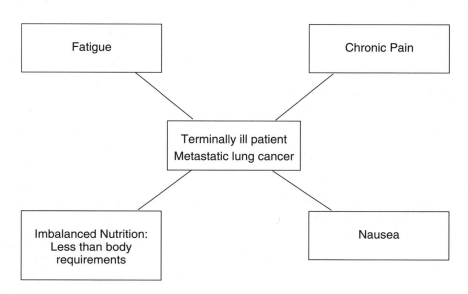

→ • Still in the chart, review the **Patient Education** notes.

4. Explain the purpose for educating the patient about mouth care.

5. Consider what you know about Pablo Rodriguez. Listed below are nonpharmacologic pain-relief interventions that may or may not be appropriate in helping Pablo Rodriguez obtain pain relief. Provide a rationale to explain why or why not to use each of the therapies for Pablo Rodriguez at this time.

Progressive relaxation

Back rub

Removing pain stimuli

Music

6. Pablo Rodriguez reports that his pain is aggravated by pressure from positioning. What intervention might you try?

Exercise 3

  CD-ROM Activity

 30 minutes

In this exercise you will visit Piya Jordan, a 68-year-old Asian-American female who entered the hospital after an emergency department admission for abdominal pain, nausea, and vomiting. She underwent abdominal surgery for the removal of a mass in her right lower quadrant. You may have worked with Piya Jordan previously if you already completed Lesson 7, 10, 14, or 15.

- Sign in to work at Pacific View Regional Hospital on the Medical-Surgical Floor for Period of Care 1. (*Note:* If you are already in the virtual hospital from a previous exercise, click on **Leave the Floor** and then **Restart the Program** to get to the sign-in window.)
- From the Patient List, select Piya Jordan (Room 403).
- Click on **Get Report**.
- Click on **Go to Nurses' Station**.
- Click on **Chart**.
- Select the chart for Room **403**.
- Click on and review the **History and Physical**.

1. After reviewing the History and Physical and the description of Piya Jordan's pain, how would you critique the quality of the physician's pain assessment? Explain.

 • Now review the **Nursing Admission**, specifically the Comfort section near the end of the form.

2. What characteristics of pain are missing from the Nursing Admission description?

 • Click on **Return to Nurses' Station**.
- Click on **EPR**.
- Click on **Login**.
- Specify **403** as the patient's room and **Vital Signs** as the category.
- Review the pain assessment.

3. Based on the data from the EPR, Piya Jordan is experiencing acute postoperative incisional pain. Her clinical summary reported restlessness and confusion from an overdose of meperidine through her PCA. What would be the priority nursing measure to initiate?
    a. Increase the dosing interval for administration of meperidine
    b. Initiate more frequent vital signs, including pain assessment
    c. Reeducate Piya Jordan and her daughter about the proper way to self-administer PCA doses
    d. Stop the PCA infusion and consult with MD about changing drug in PCA and treating patient for side effects

 • Click on **Exit EPR** and then on **Return to Nurses' Station**.
   • Click on **403** to enter Piya Jordan's room.
   • Review the **Initial Observations**.
   • Click on **Patient Care**.
   • Click on the **Nurse-Client Interactions**.
   • Select and view the video titled **0735: Pain—Adverse Drug Event Interaction**. (*Note:* If this video is not available, check the virtual clock to see whether enough time has elapsed. The video cannot be viewed before its specified time.)

4. Nonpharmacologic pain-relief interventions can be appropriate for patients in acute pain. What do you know about Piya Jordan that might make nonpharmacologic interventions appealing?

5. The Nursing Admission summary noted that Piya Jordan used a heating pad at home for pain relief. A heating pad provides pain relief through which action?
    a. Biofeedback
    b. Distraction
    c. Reducing pain perception
    d. Cutaneous stimulation

6. Piya Jordan was reported at 0700 to have confusion and restlessness. Would use of a heating pad have been appropriate for pain relief at that time? Explain.

7. Pretend that a nurse assistant who is helping you care for Piya Jordan comes to you in the hallway and says, "The patient told me she is having pain. She said it was a 7." What would you do?
    a. Go to Piya Jordan and assess the severity and character of her pain and assess her wound.
    b. Prepare an analgesic and then go to Piya Jordan's room.
    c. Prepare an analgesic and notify the physician that the patient's pain has increased.
    d. Go to Piya Jordan and assess the severity and character of her pain.

Nutrition

ᴏᴏ **Reading Assignment:** Nutrition (Chapter 31)

Patients: Jacquline Catanazaro, Medical-Surgical Floor, Room 402
Pablo Rodriguez, Medical-Surgical Floor, Room 405

Objectives:

- Compute a BMI for a patient in a case study.
- Identify the function of select nutrients.
- Describe factors that place patients at risk for nutritional problems.
- Conduct a dietary history.
- Identify clinical signs of nutritional alterations.
- Identify appropriate diet therapies for patients in the case studies.

One of the basic needs that you as a nurse must provide your patients is well-balanced, appropriate nutrition. Without adequate nutrition a patient will not have normal immune function or growth, proper wound healing or energy levels, or normal metabolic function. Many factors can affect a patient's willingness and ability to eat as a result of illness or injury. Thus, it becomes your responsibility to know how physiologic alterations affect a patient's ability to take in and digest food, factors that alter the patient's appetite, and the effects of therapeutic diet regimens. Anticipating a patient's nutritional needs can be very effective in preventing many complications of disease. In some illnesses, such as type 1 diabetes mellitus or mild hypertension, diet therapy may be the major treatment for disease control. The patient must be an active partner in helping to select meal plans and approaches that will promote or enhance nutritional intake.

Exercise 1

 CD-ROM Activity

 30 minutes

 In this exercise you will visit Jacquline Catanazaro, a 45-year-old Caucasian female who has a 30-year history of asthma, complicated by schizophrenia. She has been admitted to the emergency department because of an acute asthma episode and concurrent schizophrenic episode. You may have worked with Jacqline Catanazaro previously if you already completed Lesson 9.

- Sign in to work at Pacific View Regional Hospital on the Medical-Surgical Floor for Period of Care 1. (*Note:* If you are already in the virtual hospital from a previous exercise, click on **Leave the Floor** and then **Restart the Program** to get to the sign-in window.)
- From the Patient List, select Jacquline Catanazaro (Room 402).
- Click on **Get Report**.
- Click on **Go to Nurses' Station**.
- Click on **Chart**.
- Select the chart for Room **402**.
- Click on the **Nursing Admission**.

1. Based on your review of the information in the Nursing Admission, complete the following dietary history.

Height:	Weight:
History of food allergies:	
Number of meals per day:	
Food preferences:	
Food preparation practices:	
Appetite:	
History of weight change:	
Condition of oral cavity:	
Bowel elimination:	

2. Compute Jacquline Catanazaro's BMI. (*Study Tip:* There are 2.2 pounds in a kilogram; 1 meter equals 39.37 inches.)

3. Does Jacquline Catanazaro's BMI confirm the admission history report that the patient is obese?

➡ • Click on and review the patient's **History and Physical**.
   • Review **Consultations**, specifically the Psychiatric Consult.

4. Which of the following factors most likely has contributed to Jacquline Catanazaro's loss of appetite for the last week? (Place an X next to all that apply.)

_____ a. Albuterol

_____ b. Anxiety

_____ c. Loxapine

_____ d. Shortness of breath

_____ e. Excessive sleep

Fill in the blanks in the following statements regarding food nutrients.

5. _____ are the most calorie-dense nutrients.

6. The main source of energy in the diet is _____.

7. Based on the Food Guide Pyramid in your textbook, Jacquline Catanazaro should eat

   _____ servings of vegetables daily.

8. A regular diet includes _____ restrictions.

9. Jacquline Catanazaro's constipation might be relieved by an increase in fruits, vegetables,

   and _____.

10. Once Jacquline Catanazaro is discharged, what would be an appropriate approach for assessing her nutritional intake?

11. Following your review of the medical record, list three interventions you might use to improve Jacquline Catanazaro's nutritional status.

Exercise 2

 CD-ROM Activity

 30 minutes

 In this exercise you will visit Pablo Rodriguez, a 71-year-old Hispanic male who is suffering from advanced-stage lung cancer. You may have worked with Pablo Rodriguez previously if you already completed Lesson 4, 6, 7, 12, or 19.

- Sign in to work at Pacific View Regional Hospital on the Medical-Surgical Floor for Period of Care 2. (*Note:* If you are already in the virtual hospital from a previous exercise, click on **Leave the Floor** and then **Restart the Program** to get to the sign-in window.)
- From the Patient List, select Pablo Rodriguez (Room 405).
- Click on **Get Report**.
- Click on **Go to Nurses' Station**.
- Click on **Chart**.
- Select the chart for Room **405**.
- Click on the **Nursing Admission**.
- Click on and review the **History and Physical**.

1. List three factors that may contribute to Pablo Rodriguez's loss of appetite.

2. Match each nursing diagnosis with its cluster of defining characteristics.

Nursing Diagnosis	Defining Characteristics
_____ Nausea	a. Sore buccal cavity, aversion to eating, body weight 20% below ideal, poor muscle tone
_____ Imbalanced Nutrition: Less Than Body Requirements	b. Metallic taste, aversion to food, reports feeling of nausea
_____ Chronic Pain	c. Weight change, changes in sleep pattern, fatigue, loss of appetite

3. Is Pablo Rodriguez a candidate for enteral feeding? Explain.

4. Pablo Rodriguez has received chemotherapy and radiation, both of which can affect a patient's immune system. His loss of 50 lb over a year and his current symptoms indicate malnutrition. Malnutrition can cause which of the following?
   a. Increased skin density
   b. Shorter time for activation of lymphocytes
   c. Reduced antibodies
   d. Increased T cell formation

5. Based on your chart review, which of the following physical findings could be related to Pablo Rodriguez's nutritional status? (Place an X next to all that apply.)

   _____ a. Mild swelling of lower extremities

   _____ b. Skin warm and dry

   _____ c. No accessory muscle use

   _____ d. Swollen red gums

   _____ e. Capillary refill greater than 4 seconds

   _____ f. General muscle weakness

6. Assume that you have been successful in controlling Pablo Rodriguez's nausea and vomiting. Describe three approaches you could use to improve his appetite.

14

Elimination

Reading Assignment: Urinary Elimination (Chapter 32)
Bowel Elimination (Chapter 33)

Patients: Piya Jordan, Medical-Surgical Floor, Room 403
Jacquline Catanazaro, Medical-Surgical Floor, Room 402

Objectives:

- Describe factors that influence normal defecation.
- Describe factors that influence normal urination.
- Collect a nursing history of a patient's elimination status in a case study.
- Develop a plan of care for a patient with a bowel elimination alteration.
- Identify nursing interventions used to manage bowel elimination problems.
- Describe principles used in the care of an indwelling urinary catheter.
- Describe nursing interventions designed to reduce the risk for urinary tract infection.

Normal elimination of fecal and urinary wastes is essential for good health. When the urinary system fails to function normally, all body systems can become affected. Alterations in bowel elimination are often early signs and symptoms of problems within the gastrointestinal or other body systems. In addition, patients may experience emotional upset from having elimination alterations.

Elimination patterns and habits vary among individuals. Thus, as a nurse, you must assess any elimination problems thoroughly while applying knowledge of anatomy and physiology of the urinary and bowel systems. Thoughtful critical thinking will allow you to identify patients' problems accurately and to select relevant nursing interventions.

Exercise 1

 CD-ROM Activity

 60 minutes

 In this exercise you will visit Piya Jordan, a 68-year-old Asian-American female who entered the hospital after an emergency department admission for abdominal pain, nausea, and vomiting. She underwent abdominal surgery for the removal of a mass in her right lower quadrant. You may have worked with Piya Jordan previously if you already completed Lesson 7, 10, 12, or 15.

- Sign in to work at Pacific View Regional Hospital on the Medical-Surgical Floor for Period of Care 1. (*Note:* If you are already in the virtual hospital from a previous exercise, click on **Leave the Floor** and then **Restart the Program** to get to the sign-in window.)
- From the Patient List, select Piya Jordan (Room 403).
- Click on **Get Report**.
- Click on **Go to Nurses' Station**.
- Click on **Chart**.
- Select the chart for Room **403**.
- Click on and review the **History and Physical**.
- Click on **Diagnostic Reports** and review the summary of the abdominal CT.
- Next, click on and review the **Physician's Notes**.

1. Piya Jordan's H&P reports that she had ribbonlike stool and blood. Explain the source of these symptoms.

2. Based on your review of the abdominal CT summary, removal of Piya Jordan's mass would likely cause what change in her elimination in the future? Explain.

→ • Click on and review the **Nursing Admission**.

3. As you review Piya Jordan's admission data, complete the nursing history form below.

Nursing History Summary

Usual urinary elimination pattern:

Symptoms of urinary alteration:

Normal fluid intake:

History of urinary problems:

Usual bowel elimination pattern:

Symptoms of bowel elimination alteration:

Physical findings:

Exercise pattern:

Diet history:

Able to toilet independently?

---

4. Match each of the following factors with its corresponding effect on bowel elimination.

Factor	Effect on Bowel Elimination
_____ Physical activity	a. Increases peristalsis
_____ Fluid intake less than 1000 mL daily	b. Decreases peristalsis
_____ High-fiber diet	c. Suppresses defecation
_____ Older adulthood	
_____ Pain	
_____ Lactose intolerance	

5. Based on your knowledge that Piya Jordan has had a colon resection, as well as your review of her elimination history, list three recommendations you would make to her to ensure normal bowel elimination once she goes home.

 • Still in the chart, review the **Physician's Orders**.

6. Piya Jordan has had a urinalysis ordered for which of the following reasons?
   a. It is needed as a preoperative screening.
   b. Her intravenous infusion contains potassium.
   c. Her past history of diabetes mellitus suggests there may be glucose in her urine.
   d. She is at risk for infection because of the presence of the urinary catheter.

7. Piya Jordan has a history of stress incontinence and urgency. For each of the interventions listed below, provide a rationale.

Intervention	Rationale
a. Before discharge have patient practice how to perform pelvic floor exercises	
b. Initiate a toilet schedule on awakening	
c. Minimize the intake of tea and cola	
d. Practice deep breathing and have patient read when voiding	

8. Piya Jordan has a urinary catheter in place. On the diagram below, place an arrow at each site where introduction of infectious organisms might enter a urinary drainage system.

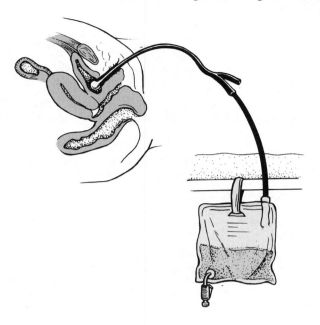

 • Click on **Return to Nurses' Station**.
• Click on Room **403** at the bottom of the screen.
• Review the **Initial Observations.**
• Click on **Patient Care**.

9. In the left column below, list the physical assessment categories you would select to perform a focused assessment of the function and effects of Piya Jordan's urinary catheter. For each category, provide a rationale for your selection.

Categories to Assess   **Rationale**

 • Based on your answer to question 9, perform the focused assessment on Piya Jordan by clicking on the appropriate categories and subcategories.

10. During the pelvic examination, the urologic assessment included a photo of Piya Jordan's catheter and drainage system. Was the catheter and drainage system anchored and positioned correctly? Explain.

11. For each of the following outcomes resulting from urinary catheterization, identify the intervention you would provide.

Outcome	Intervention
a. Urine drains freely, clear yellow	
b. Patient develops fever; urine has a foul odor	
c. Patient complains of perineal irritation at urethra	
d. Patient denies bladder discomfort	

Exercise 2

 CD-ROM Activity

 30 minutes

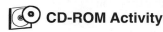 In this exercise you will meet Jacquline Catanazaro, a 45-year-old Caucasian female with a 30-year history of asthma, complicated by schizophrenia. She has been admitted to the ED because of an acute asthma episode and concurrent schizophrenic episode. You may have worked with Jacquline Catanazaro previously if you completed Lesson 9 or 13.

- Sign in to work at Pacific View Regional Hospital on the Medical-Surgical Floor for Period of Care 2. (*Note:* If you are already in the virtual hospital from a previous exercise, click on **Leave the Floor** and then **Restart the Program** to get to the sign-in window.)
- From the Patient List, select Jacquline Catanazaro (Room 402).
- Click on **Get Report**.
- Click on **Go to Nurses' Station**.
- Click on **Chart**.
- Select the chart for Room **402**.
- Click on **Nursing Admission** and review.

1. Place an X next to all factors contributing to Jacquline Catanazaro's bowel elimination problems.

    _____ a. Physical inactivity

    _____ b. Age

    _____ c. Emotional stress

    _____ d. Limited intake of high-fiber foods

    _____ e. Reduced fluid intake

    _____ f. Obesity

2. Jacquline Catanazaro's Nursing Admission states that she reports a pattern of a bowel movement every 1 to 2 days and perceives having constipation. She also reports a hard stool. What two additional symptoms might you assess to confirm constipation for this patient?

 • Click on **Return to Nurses' Station**.
- Click on **402** to enter the patient's room.
- Review the **Initial Observations**.
- Click on **Patient Care**.
- Click on **Abdomen**.
- Review the examination of the abdomen.

3. Jacquline Catanazaro exhibited the physical findings listed below. Next to each finding, describe what you would more likely find if the patient had constipation.

Physical Finding	Constipation Finding
a. Abdomen soft and flat	
b. Bowel sounds normal	
c. No abdominal tenderness or masses	

- Click on **Nurse-Client Interactions**.
- Select and view the video titled **1140: Compliance—Medications**. (*Note:* If this video is not available, check the virtual clock to see whether enough time has elapsed. The video cannot be viewed before its specified time.)

4. Jacquline Catanazaro's Nursing Admission and the video reveal the following three data clusters. Identify the nursing diagnosis for each cluster. (*Study Tip:* Refer to a resource for NANDA nursing diagnoses.)

Data Cluster	Nursing Diagnosis

a. Emotional stress
  Insufficient fiber intake
  Poor eating habits;
    does not eat vegetables or fruits
  Insufficient fluid intake
  Antipsychotic/sedative use	

b. Dysfunctional eating pattern,
    4 to 6 meals a day
  Sedentary activity level
  Weight 20% over ideal for height	

c. Inability to take responsibility for
    meeting health practices; does
    not remember to take medications
  Lack of adaptive behavior to
    environmental changes; anxious
    and agitated
  Lack of knowledge regarding health
    practices; "It takes a lot for me to
    remember"	

5. Consider how the nursing diagnoses you identified in question 4 are interrelated. Below, develop a plan of care for the nursing diagnosis Risk for Constipation.

Nursing Diagnosis: Risk for Constipation

Goal

Outcomes

Interventions

Rationales

6. Assume that the nurse decided to consult with the physician about ordering a medication for Jacquline Catanazaro. What might be the best recommendation to relieve her constipation? Explain.

7. If you were the nurse caring for Jacquline Catanazaro 2 days after initiating treatment for constipation, what evaluation measures would you use to determine whether the plan of care was effective?

LESSON 15

Care of the Surgical Patient

ᴓᴅ **Reading Assignment:** Surgical Patient (Chapter 37)
Skin Integrity and Wound Care (Chapter 35)

Patient: Piya Jordan, Medical-Surgical Floor, Room 403

Objectives:

1. Describe criteria to use in the preoperative assessment of a surgical patient.
2. Explain the rationale for postoperative exercises.
3. Discuss principles to incorporate in a preoperative teaching plan.
4. Describe risks for postoperative complications in case study patients.
5. Identify risks associated with different forms of anesthesia.
6. Apply critical thinking to the assessment of a postoperative patient.
7. Identify signs and symptoms of common postoperative complications.
8. Describe nursing interventions for preventing postoperative complications.

Perioperative nursing care is the care administered before (preoperative), during (intraoperative) and after (postoperative) surgery. Because surgery occurs in both outpatient and inpatient settings, a surgical nurse must be able to anticipate patients' risks for problems, know the anticipated effects of surgery, recognize early signs of complications, and know how to intervene in all situations. Patients who undergo surgery become dependent on the nurse for physical as well as psychological comfort. However, when patients become active participants in their preoperative and postoperative care, the incidence of complications is less likely. Thorough preoperative education is essential to ensure appropriate and safe care for the surgical patient.

Exercise 1

 CD-ROM Activity

 45 minutes

 In this exercise you will visit Piya Jordan, a 68-year-old Asian-American female who entered the hospital after an emergency department admission for abdominal pain, nausea, and vomiting. She underwent abdominal surgery for the removal of a mass in her right lower quadrant. You may have worked with Piya Jordan previously if you already completed Lesson 7, 10, 12, or 14.

- Sign in to work at Pacific View Regional Hospital on the Medical-Surgical Floor for Period of Care 1. (*Note:* If you are already in the virtual hospital from a previous exercise, click on **Leave the Floor** and then **Restart the Program** to get to the sign-in window.)
- From the Patient List, select Piya Jordan (Room 403).
- Click on **Get Report**.
- Click on **Go to Nurses' Station**.
- Click on **Chart**.
- Click on the chart for Room **403**.
- Review the **Nursing Admission**.

1. Based on the Nursing Admission data, place an X next to the surgical risk factors below that apply to Piya Jordan.

    _____ a. Obesity

    _____ b. Heart disease

    _____ c. Fever

    _____ d. Nutritional imbalance

    _____ e. Chronic pain

    _____ f. Age

    _____ g. Liver disease

2. Identify two alterations of the cardiovascular system that may apply to Piya Jordan because of her age.

- Click on and review the **History and Physical**.
- Click on and review the **Laboratory Results**.

3. The physician's History and Physical noted the need to correct Piya Jordan's electrolytes and reverse anticoagulation prior to surgery. Which laboratory values were abnormal in Piya Jordan's case? (Place an X next to all that apply.)

_____ a. RBC

_____ b. INR

_____ c. Potassium

_____ d. Sodium

_____ e. Hgb

_____ f. Creatinine

4. Give a reason for why you think Piya Jordan's Hgb and RBC values were lower than normal prior to surgery. Why are changes in these lab values significant?

5. What is the most likely reason that Piya Jordan's INR is higher than normal?
   a. Inflammation of her knee joints
   b. Warfarin therapy at home
   c. Irregular nature of her heart rate
   d. Blood in her stool

6. Because of the elevated INR, Piya Jordan would be at risk for which of the following complications during surgery?
   a. Urinary retention
   b. Pneumonia
   c. Paralytic ileus
   d. Hemorrhage

 • Still in the chart, click again on **Nursing Admission** and review the summaries for Perception & Cognition, Self-Perception, Role Relationships, and Coping.

• Now review the **Nurse's Notes** from Tuesday 0330 to Tuesday 0900.

7. The nurse's assessment should focus on factors that will influence the ability to provide Piya Jordan with preoperative instruction. Listed below are numerous factors identified in Piya Jordan's assessment. Complete this exercise by indicating whether each factor would facilitate instruction (positive) or would be a barrier to instruction (negative).

Assessment Factor	Effect on Instruction
_____ Patient reports a pain score of 8 out of 10	a. Positive
_____ Patient expresses being anxious about husband's welfare	b. Negative
_____ Daughter is supportive of mother	
_____ Patient is fearful of cancer diagnosis	
_____ Patient speaks English and has college education	
_____ Patient reports feeling nauseated	

8. Based on information from the Nurse's Notes and Nursing Admission, what would be the best time to teach Piya Jordan about deep breathing and coughing exercises? Give a rationale.

9. After surgery, it is important to turn patients frequently. What factor in Piya Jordan's history might make turning difficult for her?

10. Match the preoperative exercises with the postoperative complications they prevent. Each exercise can have more than one answer.

Preoperative Exercise	Postoperative Complication
_____ Deep breathing	a. Pneumonia
_____ Coughing	b. Thrombus formation
_____ Turning	c. Atelectasis
_____ Leg exercises	d. Joint immobility
_____ Incentive spirometry	

Exercise 2

 CD-ROM Activity

 30 minutes

 In this exercise you will visit Piya Jordan, a 68-year-old Asian-American female who entered the hospital after an emergency department admission for abdominal pain, nausea, and vomiting. She underwent abdominal surgery for the removal of a mass in her right lower quadrant. You may have worked with Piya Jordan previously if you already completed Lesson 7, 10, 12, or 14.

- Sign in to work at Pacific View Regional Hospital on the Medical-Surgical Floor for Period of Care 1. (*Note:* If you are already in the virtual hospital from a previous exercise, click on **Leave the Floor** and then **Restart the Program** to get to the sign-in window.)
- From the Patient List, select Piya Jordan (Room 403).
- Click on **Get Report**.
- Click on **Go to Nurses' Station**.
- Click on **Chart**.
- Click on the chart for Room **403**.
- Click on and review the **Nurse's Notes**.
- Next, review the **Postoperative Notes**.
- Finally, review the **Physician's Notes**.

1. For each of the interventions listed below and on the next page, give a rationale for its use in Piya Jordan's case.

Jackson-Pratt drain

Sequential compression device

Nasogastric tube

Abdominal dressing

2. Which of the following findings is abnormal in Piya Jordan's case?
   a. NG draining moderate brown drainage
   b. Telemetry showing atrial fibrillation
   c. Urine clear, dark yellow
   d. Jackson-Pratt draining serosanguinous drainage

3. After reviewing the clinical summary and the Nurse's Notes, what common postoperative complication might Piya Jordan be at risk for, unless the nurse more actively intervenes? Give a rationale and explain the interventions required.

 • Click on **Return to Nurses' Station**.
   • Select Room **403** at the bottom of the screen.
   • Click on **Patient Care**.
   • Click on **Abdomen**.
   • Review the findings of the abdominal assessment, specifically the subcategories of **Integumentary** and **Gastrointestinal**.

4. What type of dressing does Piya Jordan have over her abdomen? How is it secured?

5. What is the most critical time for healing of a surgical wound?
   a. First 24 hours postop
   b. 7 days postop
   c. 24 to 72 hours postop
   d. 15 to 20 days postop

• Conduct a focused physical examination of Piya Jordan by clicking on the various yellow assessment buttons and green subcategories as needed based on your answer to question 6.

6. As the nurse caring for Piya Jordan postoperatively, you would want to do a focused assessment when you begin your care. Which assessment categories would you select to focus on her postoperative status? (*Hint:* Do not forget to assess equipment.)

 • When you have completed your focused assessment, click on **Leave the Floor**.
• From the Floor Menu, choose **Look at Your Preceptor's Evaluation**.
• Next, click on **Examination Report** to see how you did.

Exercise 3

 CD-ROM Activity

 45 minutes

 In this exercise you will visit Piya Jordan, a 68-year-old Asian-American female who entered the hospital after an emergency department admission for abdominal pain, nausea, and vomiting. She underwent abdominal surgery for the removal of a mass in her right lower quadrant. You may have worked with Piya Jordan previously if you already completed Lesson 7, 10, 12, or 14.

• Sign in to work at Pacific View Regional Hospital on the Medical-Surgical Floor for Period of Care 2. (*Note:* If you are already in the virtual hospital from a previous exercise, click on **Leave the Floor** and then **Restart the Program** to get to the sign-in window.)
• From the Patient List, select Piya Jordan (Room 403).
• Click on **Get Report**.
• Click on **Go to Nurses' Station**.
• Click on **Chart**.
• Click on the chart for Room **403**.
• Review the **Nursing Admission**.
• Review the **Surgical Reports**.

1. Considering the type of anesthesia Piya Jordan received, she is most at risk for which of the following?
   a. Respiratory depression, cardiovascular irritability, and liver damage
   b. Respiratory paralysis and hypotension
   c. Loss of sensation and pain reception in operative area
   d. Headache, urinary retention, and back pain

 • Click on **Nurse's Notes** and review the notes for Wednesday at 1115.
   • Click on **Return to Nurses' Station**.
   • Select Room **403** at the bottom of the screen.
   • Review the **Initial Observations**.
   • Click on **Patient Care**.
   • Click on **Nurse-Client Interactions**.
   • Select and view the video titled **1115: Interventions—Nausea, Blood**. (*Note:* If this video is not available, check the virtual clock to see whether enough time has elapsed. The video cannot be viewed before its specified time.)

2. Piya Jordan is complaining of nausea. What is the likely source of the nausea?

3. Identify three assessments necessary to determine the source and nature of Piya Jordan's nausea.

4. When an NG tube's patency is in question, what is the appropriate action?
   a. Remove the tube from suction and call the physician
   b. Irrigate the tube with normal saline
   c. Reposition the tube
   d. Obtain an x-ray of the abdomen

 • Click on **Physical Assessment**.
   • Click on **Chest** and then on the appropriate subcategories to review the assessment of Piya Jordan's chest.
   • Next, click on **Abdomen** and the related subcategories to review the abdominal assessment.
   • Now click on **Take Vital Signs** at the top of the screen.

5. After reviewing the data available on Piya Jordan, clusters of data are revealed from the assessment. One data cluster for this patient is listed below:

> Chest expansion decreased
> Decreased aeration, both lower lobes
> Patient has had acute pain
> Abdomen tender to palpation
> Has not used incentive spirometer

What potential problem/nursing diagnosis is indicated by this data cluster?

6. A nurse who has cared for Piya Jordan tells you that one of her nursing diagnoses is Risk for Infection. Give a rationale for why this diagnosis would apply to Piya Jordan.

7. Piya Jordan has several problems resulting from her postoperative condition and concern regarding cancer. Develop a concept map by drawing arrows to show the association between three of those nursing diagnoses. (*Study Tip:* See pages 121-122 in your textbook.)

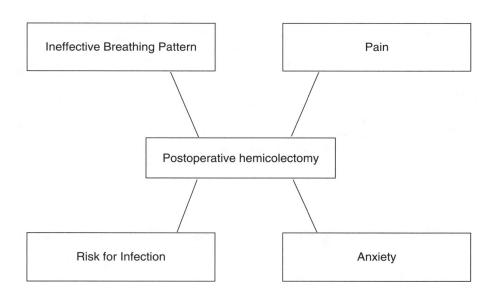

8. Complete the plan of care below for the nursing diagnosis Ineffective Breathing Pattern.

Nursing Diagnosis: Ineffective Breathing Pattern

Goal

Expected Outcomes

Interventions

1.

2.

3.

4.

Evaluation Measures

1.

2.

3.

Wound Care

Reading Assignment: Skin Integrity and Wound Care (Chapter 35)

Patients: Harry George, Medical-Surgical Floor, Room 401
Goro Oishi, Skilled Nursing Floor, Room 505

Objectives:

- Describe risk factors contributing to pressure ulcer formation.
- Use a pressure ulcer risk assessment tool for a patient in a case study.
- Explain factors that slow or promote wound healing.
- Identify types of wounds.
- Describe characteristics of a wound.
- Identify interventions used in the prevention of pressure ulcers.
- Explain the purpose of a wound dressing.
- Discuss factors to consider in selecting a wound dressing.
- Describe steps used in the application of dressings.

The skin is a protective barrier against disease-causing organisms, and it is a sensory organ for pain, temperature and touch. A break in skin integrity resulting from pressure, trauma, or surgical intervention creates a risk for patients, especially those with impaired wound healing. Good wound care practices involve active prevention. For example, a patient at risk for developing a pressure ulcer should be routinely mobilized or repositioned and given the appropriate type of skin care. A patient with a surgical wound requires meticulous wound care to prevent infection. As a nurse, you should know the risks associated with skin breakdown and the normal processes of wound healing to enable you to provide safe and appropriate care to your patients.

Exercise 1

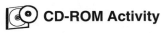 **CD-ROM Activity**

 45 minutes

 In this exercise you will visit Harry George, a 42-year-old Caucasian male who was admitted to the hospital with symptoms of infection and swelling of the foot. He has a history of abusing alcohol. He has been diagnosed with cellulitis and osteomyelitis of the foot. You may have worked with Harry George previously if you already completed Lesson 1 or 18.

- Sign in to work at Pacific View Regional Hospital on the Medical-Surgical Floor for Period of Care 1. (*Note:* If you are already in the virtual hospital from a previous exercise, click on **Leave the Floor** and then **Restart the Program** to get to the sign-in window.)
- From the Patient List, select Harry George (Room 401).
- Click on **Get Report**.
- Click on **Go to Nurses' Station**.
- Click on **Chart**.
- Select the chart for Room **401**.
- Review the **Nursing Admission**.
- Next, review the **History and Physical**.

1. Listed below are factors that influence wound healing. Place an X next to all of the factors that apply to Harry George.

_____ a. Nutrition

_____ b. Smoking

_____ c. Circulation

_____ d. Drugs

_____ e. Obesity

_____ f. Infection

_____ g. Age

_____ h. Wound stress

_____ i. Diabetes

2. Provide a rationale for why each of the following factors affects wound healing.

Circulation

Diabetes

Smoking

3. Based on the description of Harry George's wound, the type of drainage can best be described as:
   a. thick, yellow or brown.
   b. clear, watery plasma.
   c. pale, red, watery.
   d. bright red.

 • Click on **Return to Nurses' Station**.
 • Click on Room **401** at the bottom of the screen.
 • Read the **Initial Observations** of Harry George's status.

4. Explain why Harry George's left foot is elevated.

 • Next, click on **Patient Care**.
 • Select **Lower Extremities** and review each of the four subcategories for assessment findings.

 5. Good wound assessment requires the use of appropriate physical assessment techniques. (*Study Tip:* Review Chapter 13 in your textbook for techniques.) Match the physical assessment findings on the left with the assessment techniques on the right.

	Physical Finding	**Assessment Technique**
_____	Wound draining serous drainage	a. Inspection
_____	Posterior tibial pulse 1+ on left	b. Palpation
_____	Skin warm and dry	c. Measurement
_____	Open lesion 2-3 centimeters	
_____	Capillary refill sluggish	
_____	Erythema over anterior tibia	

6. Refer to the wound classifications on page 1019 in your textbook. Using this information, what stage would you use to describe Harry George's wound?

 • Click on **Chart**.
• Select the chart for Room **401**.
• Click on **History and Physical** and review, specifically the Social History section.

7. What factor(s) in Harry George's social history may be implicated in his ability to care for his wound? Explain.

 • Now review the **Physician's Notes**.
• Next, click on **Consultations** and review the wound care team summary note.

8. The wound care note describes Harry George's dressing as occlusive. Which of the following dressings is most likely being used for Harry George?
a. Wet to dry
b. Telfa gauze
c. Hydrocolloid
d. Foam dressing

9. Give a rationale for your answer to question 8.

10. List three nursing actions that are important when preparing a patient for a dressing change.

True or False. Select true or false for questions 11 through 14.

11. Hydrocolloid dressings support would healing by debriding necrotic wounds.
    a. True
    b. False

12. Hydrogel dressings can absorb large amounts of exudate.
    a. True
    b. False

13. Before removing a wet-to-dry dressing, you should moisten the dressing with saline.
    a. True
    b. False

14. When selecting a dressing, you should choose one that keeps the surrounding intact skin dry.
    a. True
    b. False

Exercise 2

 CD-ROM Activity

 45 minutes

 In this exercise you will visit Goro Oishi, a 66-year-old Asian-American male who is admitted for hospice care following an intracerebral hemorrhage. You may have worked with Goro Oishi previously if you already completed Lesson 8 or 17.

- Sign in to work at Pacific View Regional Hospital on the Skilled Nursing Floor for Period of Care 1. (*Note:* If you are already in the virtual hospital from a previous exercise, click on **Leave the Floor** and then **Restart the Program** to get to the sign-in window.)
- From the Patient List, select Goro Oishi (Room 505).
- Click on **Get Report**.
- Click on **Go to Nurses' Station**.
- Click on **Chart**.
- Select the chart for Room **505**.
- Review the **Nursing Admission**.

1. Place an X next to the current risk factors for Goro Oishi to develop a pressure ulcer.

    _____ a. Impaired sensation

    _____ b. Impaired mobility

    _____ c. Altered level of consciousness

    _____ d. Moisture

2. What would be Goro Oishi's Braden Scale score? (*Study Tip:* See page 1023 in your textbook.)

3. What intervention is most likely preventing prolonged exposure of Goro Oishi's skin to moisture?

• Click on **Return to Nurses' Station**.
• Click on **505** to enter Goro Oishi's room.
• Review the **Initial Observations**.
• Click on **Patient Care**.
• Review assessment of the integument for each of the physical assessment categories. (*Hint:* First click on **Head & Neck** and select **Integumentary** from the list of subcategories. Next, click on **Chest** and then on **Integumentary**. Continue until you have reviewed the Integumentary assessments in all seven body areas.)

4. In the diagram below, place an X in each of the circles where Goro Oishi is at risk for a pressure ulcer to form.

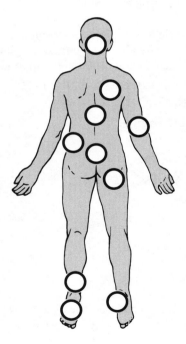

• Click on **EPR** and then on **Login**.
- Specify **505** as the patient's room and **Integumentary** as the category.
- Review the flow sheet data for the integument.
- Now change the category to **Hygiene and Comfort** and review this flow sheet.

5. Goro Oishi's Braden Scale score indicates that he is at high risk for a pressure ulcer to develop. List three interventions for a high-risk ulcer prevention protocol.

6. Answer the following questions based on your review of the EPR data.

   a. Do you believe Goro Oishi is being turned often enough?

   b. What time is he due to be turned again on the current schedule?

   c. In what position should he be placed?

   d. What specialty mattress is currently in use?

7. Which of the following are correct interventions the nurse should perform each time Goro Oishi is turned? (Place an X next to all that apply.)

   _____ a. Assess the area the patient was previously lying over for redness.

   _____ b. Massage any area of redness.

   _____ c. Check underlying linen for moisture.

   _____ d. Apply additional moisturizer to the skin.

8. If you were selecting a support surface on which to place Goro Oishi, what type would you choose? Give a rationale.

 • Click on **Exit EPR**.
• Click on **Nurses' Station**.
• Click on **Chart**.
• Select the chart for Room **505**.
• Review the **Nurse's Notes**.

9. Goro Oishi is currently receiving IV fluids. The change in nutritional therapy recommended by the physician will provide what benefit?

LESSON **17**

Loss and Grief and Nursing Interventions to Support Coping

Reading Assignment: Stress and Coping (Chapter 22)
                             Loss and Grief (Chapter 23)

Patients: Goro Oishi, Skilled Nursing Floor, Room 505
                 Harry George, Medical-Surgical Floor, Room 401

Objectives:

- Describe types of loss.
- Describe loss and grief responses of patients and families in the case studies.
- Identify characteristics of a person experiencing grief.
- Explain the relationship between loss and stress.
- Describe coping mechanisms used by patients in the case studies.
- Describe the use of hope in support of a patient in grief.
- Describe principles of palliative care.
- Identify nursing diagnoses applicable to a patient requiring palliative care.
- Develop a concept map for a patient facing death.

Loss and grief are experiences that affect patients, families, and caregivers alike. You probably entered the nursing profession to help patients recover from illness or to achieve an improved level of health. Your knowledge, experience, and skill cannot always result in cure for your patients.

Patients and their families can experience loss and grief in many forms. It is important for a patient to be able to experience and express grief in order to achieve healing. As a nurse, you are responsible for assisting patients to feel and express their loss and to find realistic and relevant ways for coping. In cases where patients face long-term chronic or terminal illness, palliative care becomes essential. Palliative care includes preventive and supportive interventions designed to help patients approach the end of their life. Understanding grief and loss, the concepts of coping, and the principles of palliative care will prepare you to give skilled and compassionate care to those patients who face loss and death.

Exercise 1

 CD-ROM Activity

 60 minutes

In this exercise you will visit Goro Oishi, a 66-year-old Asian-American male who is admitted for hospice care following an intracerebral hemorrhage. You may have worked with this patient previously if you already completed Lesson 8 or 16.

- Sign in to work at Pacific View Regional Hospital on the Skilled Nursing Floor for Period of Care 1. (*Note:* If you are already in the virtual hospital from a previous exercise, click on **Leave the Floor** and then **Restart the Program** to get to the sign-in window.)
- From the Patient List, select Goro Oishi (Room 505).
- Click on **Get Report**.
- Click on **Go to Nurses' Station**.
- Click on **Chart**.
- Click on the chart for Room **505**.
- Review the **Nursing Admission**.

1. Goro Oishi has been admitted for hospice care. Which of the following describe the components or features of a hospice care program? (Place an X next to all that apply.)

    _____ a. A facility for treatment of terminal illnesses

    _____ b. Treatment philosophy focused on symptom control

    _____ c. Interdisciplinary care team approach

    _____ d. Care providers set goals made to meet the family's desires

    _____ e. Coordination of home care services

2. Patients experience different types of loss.

    a. Based on the Nursing Admission summary of role relationships, identify the type of loss Goro Oishi experienced just prior to his stroke and explain its significance.

    b. How did Goro Oishi choose to cope with his loss?

➡ • Review the **Physician's Notes**.
  • Next, review the **Nurse's Notes**.

3. The notes state that Goro Oishi's family feels conflicted about whether or not to initiate enteral feeding. Which of the stages of grief below might describe the family's response? (Place an X next to all that apply.)

_____ a. Adjusting to the environment without the deceased

_____ b. Reorganization

_____ c. Denial

_____ d. Bargaining

_____ e. Emotionally relocating the deceased

➡ • Click on **Return to Nurses' Station**.
  • Click on Room **505** at the bottom of the screen.
  • Read the **Initial Observations.**
  • Click on **Patient Care**.
  • Click on **Nurse-Client Interactions**.
  • Observe the following three video interactions: **0735: Assessment—Family**, **0750: Family Conflict—Plan of Care**, and **0755: Death—The Right to Die**. (*Note:* If any of these videos are not available, check the virtual clock to see whether enough time has elapsed. The videos cannot be viewed before their specified time.)

4. After considering data from the Nursing Admission and observing Goro Oishi's wife during the videos, you recognize a variety of factors influencing her perception of loss. For each of the following factors, describe the conditions affecting Mrs. Oishi's response to loss.

Nature of loss

Personal relationship

Culture

Spiritual belief

→ • Click on **Physical Assessment**.
  • Review each of the physical examination categories.

5. As you review the physical examination, also consider data from the Nursing Admission. The data you obtain begin to form patterns of information. A patient in need of palliative care has numerous health problems. Summarize your findings for each category listed below.

Skin integrity

Mobility

Respirations

Airway status

Fluid balance

6. As you begin to see patterns in Goro Oishi's data, nursing diagnoses also begin to emerge. Match the defining characteristics from the patient's database with the corresponding nursing diagnosis.

Nursing Diagnosis	Defining Characteristics
_____ Impaired Bed Mobility	a. No gag reflex
_____ Risk for Aspiration	b. Cool and pale skin
_____ Risk for Impaired Skin Integrity	c. No spontaneous movement
_____ Impaired Gas Exchange	d. Shallow respirations
	e. Unable to move limbs independently
	f. Febrile
	g. Unable to swallow
	h. Physically immobile
	i. Oxygen saturation 88%

 7. Given Goro Oishi's numerous physical problems, develop a concept map by drawing arrows to show the association between nursing diagnoses. (*Study Tip:* See pages 121-122 in your textbook.)

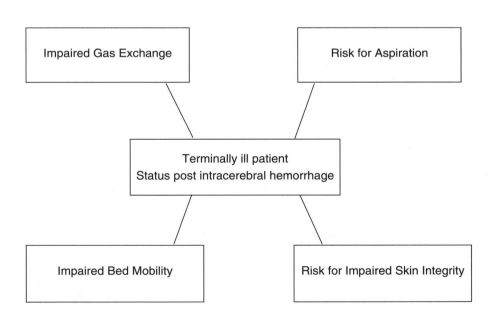

- Click on **Leave the Floor**; then click on **Restart the Program**.
- Sign in to work on the Skilled Nursing Floor, this time for Period of Care 3.
- From the Patient List, select Goro Oishi (Room 505).
- Click on **Get Report** and review. Then click on **Go to Nurses' Station**.
- Click on Room **505** at bottom of the screen.
- Review the **Initial Observations**.
- Now click on **Patient Care** and then on **Nurse-Client Interactions**.
- Select and view the video titled **1500: Patient Decline**.

8. Goro Oishi is progressively worsening. His breathing pattern is becoming more dyspneic as intracranial pressure builds from his hemorrhage. List three approaches you can use in promoting comfort for a patient with ineffective breathing patterns.

9. In the video interaction, the nurse asks Mrs. Oishi to leave the bedside momentarily, so that the nurse can speak with her. Support of the grieving family is important at this time. Identify three interventions the nurse may use to support Mrs. Oishi.

Select true or false for questions 10 through 14.

10. At the time of a patient's death, federal law requires identification of potential organ or tissue donors.
   a. True
   b. False

11. It is the nurse's responsibility to ask permission for an autopsy.
   a. True
   b. False

12. During the care of the body, after death, it is important to remove the patient's dentures.
   a. True
   b. False

13. While preparing the body, name tags are placed on the body to identify it.
   a. True
   b. False

14. At the time of death, the family must know who among them can legally give consent for organ donation.
   a. True
   b. False

Exercise 2

 CD-ROM Activity

 30 minutes

 In this exercise you will visit Harry George, a 42-year-old Caucasian male who was admitted to the hospital with symptoms of infection and swelling of the foot. He has a history of abusing alcohol. He has been diagnosed with cellulitis and osteomyelitis of the foot. You may have worked with Harry George previously if you already completed Lesson 1, 16, or 18.

- Sign in to work at Pacific View Regional Hospital on the Medical-Surgical Floor for Period of Care 1. (*Note:* If you are already in the virtual hospital from a previous exercise, click on **Leave the Floor** and then **Restart the Program** to get to the sign-in window.)
- From the Patient List, select Harry George (Room 401).
- Click on **Get Report**.
- Click on **Go to Nurses' Station**.
- Click on **Chart**.
- Select the chart for Room **406**.
- Click on and review the **Nursing Admission**.
- Now review the **History and Physical**.

1. Harry George has experienced different types of loss. Each are affected by the level of stress he has experienced. Describe a source of stress Harry George is experiencing for each of the factors below.

Situational

Maturational

Sociocultural

2. A focused assessment will help the nurse better understand the nature of stress affecting Harry George. For each of the assessment categories below, write in two questions you would ask of the patient.

Perception of stressor

Adherence to healthy practices

3. Describe both the actual and perceived losses experienced by Harry George.

Actual

Perceived

4. When assessing a patient's stage of grief, it is important for the nurse to assess how a

   patient _____ reacting rather than how the patient should be reacting.

5. A person who becomes overwhelmed by grief and often takes on self-destructive behavior

   is experiencing _____ grief.

6. According to Bowlby's phases of mourning, the phase of _____
   arouses emotional outbursts and acute distress.

7. _____ is defined as the anticipation of a continued good.

8. For each of the following dimensions, describe a nursing intervention that would realistically promote hope for Harry George.

Cognitive dimension

Behavioral dimension

Contextual dimension

LESSON 18

Self-Concept

👓 **Reading Assignment:** Self-Concept and Sexuality (Chapter 20)

Patients: Harry George, Medical-Surgical Floor, Room 401
Dorothy Grant, Obstetrics Floor, Room 201

Objectives:

- Identify the components of self-concept.
- Describe stressors that affect self-concept of patients in the case studies.
- Discuss the influence of a nurse's behavior on patients' self-concept.
- Apply the critical thinking model to assessment of a patient's self-concept.
- Develop a concept map for a case study patient with self-concept alterations.
- Describe the nursing diagnostic process for a patient with alteration in self-concept.
- Identify interventions useful in the promotion of self-concept.

The self-concept is a complex mixture of thoughts, attitudes, and perceptions that shape how a person thinks about himself or herself. A person's self-concept affects all situations and relationships with others, in addition to that person's own self-esteem. Disease, injury, and resultant disability all can threaten a person's self-concept and self-esteem. As a nurse, you play an important role in helping patients adapt to stressors caused by health alterations. What individuals think and how they feel about themselves affect the way they care for themselves physically and emotionally. Knowledge of variables that affect self-concept and of the approaches used in promoting self-concept will enable you to provide patients with appropriate support and treatment.

Exercise 1

  CD-ROM Activity

 45 minutes

In this exercise you will visit Harry George, a 42-year-old Caucasian male who was admitted to the hospital with symptoms of infection and swelling of the foot. He has a history of abusing alcohol. He has been diagnosed with cellulitis and osteomyelitis of the foot. You may have worked with Harry George previously if you already completed Lesson 1 or 16.

• Sign in to work at Pacific View Regional Hospital on the Medical-Surgical Floor for Period of Care 3. (*Note:* If you are already in the virtual hospital from a previous exercise, click on **Leave the Floor** and then **Restart the Program** to get to the sign-in window.)
• From the Patient List, select Harry George (Room 401).
• Click on **Get Report**.
• Click on **Go to Nurses' Station**.
• Click on **Chart**.
• Select the chart for Room **401**.
• First, review the **Nursing Admission** history.
• Next, review the physician's **History and Physical**.

1. Self-concept is always changing and developing. Place an X next to those factors that have affected Harry George's self-concept since his motorcycle accident 4 years ago.

_____ a. Sense of competency

_____ b. Perceived reaction of others to his body

_____ c. Employment related identity

_____ d. Perceptions of events that have affected self

_____ e. Racial identity

_____ f. Self-expectations

2. Explain how the loss of employment has likely affected Harry George's self-concept.

 3. Of the following developmental stages of life described by Erik Erikson, which is most likely disrupted in the case of Harry George? (*Study Tip:* Review Erikson's theory on page 530 in your textbook.)
a. Integrity versus despair
b. Industry versus inferiority
c. Initiative versus guilt
d. Generativity versus self-absorption and stagnation

• Now click on **Consultations**.
  • Review the Psychiatric Consult.
  • Review the Mental Health Summary.

4. A self-concept stressor threatens a person's identity, body image, and role performance. Match the stressors experienced by Harry George with the appropriate self-concept category.

Harry George's Stressors	**Self-Concept Categories**
_____ Impotence	a. Body image
_____ Loss of role as husband	b. Identity
_____ Emotional depression	c. Role performance
_____ Failure to maintain personal grooming	
_____ Job loss	
_____ Chronic wound	
_____ Seen as a public nuisance	

5. The expectations of family and friends on how Harry George should have behaved immediately following his injury would be described as a _____ role.

6. Harry George's _____ image involves attitudes he has about his appearance, impotence, and the effects of his diabetes.

7. Harry George's emotional appraisal of himself as a "loser" is a form of self-evaluation described as _____ esteem.

8. Harry George's _____ performance is the way in which he perceives his ability to be competent as a parent.

9. Making a nursing diagnosis when a patient has an alteration in self-concept is complex. Often an assessment finding can be a defining characteristic for more than one nursing diagnosis. The defining characteristics from Harry George's database are listed at the bottom of this page. Complete the concept map below by writing the letter of each defining characteristic under the appropriate nursing diagnoses. (*Note:* A defining characteristic may be used for more than one diagnosis.)

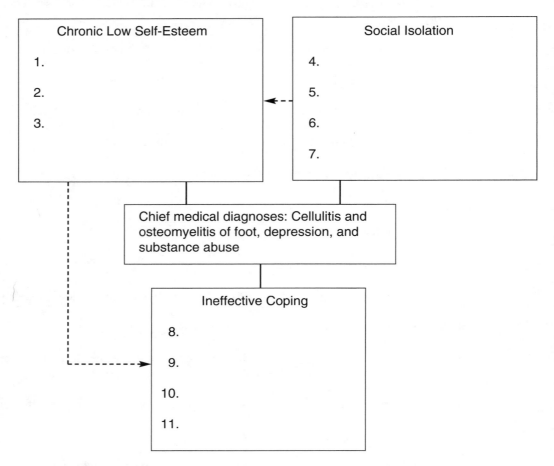

Defining Characteristics:

a. Sleep disturbance
b. Expression of shame/guilt
c. Change in communication pattern/uncommunicative
d. Abuse of chemical agent
e. Exists in a subculture
f. Inability to meet basic needs
g. Sad affect
h. Poor or no eye contact
i. Self-negating verbalization

10. Harry George is a complex case. Given the nursing diagnoses of Chronic Low Self-Esteem, Social Isolation, and Ineffective Coping, which would likely be your priority? Explain.

Exercise 2

 CD-ROM Activity

 45 minutes

 In this exercise you will visit Dorothy Grant, a pregnant 25-year-old Caucasian patient who was admitted to the hospital after blunt trauma to the abdomen. You may have worked with Dorothy Grant previously if you already completed Lesson 4.

• Sign in to work at Pacific View Regional Hospital on the Obstetrics Floor for Period of Care 1. (*Note:* If you are already in the virtual hospital from a previous exercise, click on **Leave the Floor** and then **Restart the Program** to get to the sign-in window.)
• From the Patient List, select Dorothy Grant (Room 201).
• Click on **Get Report**.
• Click on **Go to Nurses' Station**.
• Click on **Chart**.
• Select the chart for Room **201**.
• Review the **History and Physical**.
• Next, review the **Nursing Admission**.

1. As a victim of abuse, Dorothy Grant faces many factors that threaten her self-concept. Her concern for her unborn baby and children creates stress on her ability to function as a wife and mother. Application of critical thinking will ensure a more comprehensive assessment of this patient's situation. Complete the following critical thinking diagram for assessment of Dorothy Grant's situation by writing the letter of each critical thinking factor under its proper category.

Knowledge

1. _____

2. _____

3. _____

Experience	**ASSESSMENT SELF-CONCEPT**	**Attitudes**
4. _____		5. _____
		6. _____

Standards

7. _____

8. _____

9. _____

Critical Thinking Factors

a. Consider your own feelings if, as a parent, you have believed your children were at risk.
b. Ask Dorothy Grant, "You said you want to be a good mother. Tell me what you mean by that."
c. Review concepts on domestic violence.
d. While caring for Dorothy Grant, apply what you have learned in caring for other victims of abuse.
e. While assessing Dorothy Grant, reinforce that any decisions about getting help to leave her husband will be her decisions only.
f. Consider concepts about self-esteem as you assess Dorothy Grant's needs.
g. Ask Dorothy Grant to tell her story by saying, "Tell me how your relationship with your husband has changed since you first married."
h. Ask the patient if you can talk with her sister about her relationship with her children.
i. Apply principles of communication and caring while establishing a therapeutic relationship with Dorothy Grant.

- Click on **Return to Nurses' Station**.
- Click on **Leave the Floor**.
- Click on **Restart the Program**.
- Sign in to work at Pacific View Regional Hospital on the Obstetrics Floor for Period of Care 2.
- From the Patient List, select Dorothy Grant (Room 201).
- Click on **Get Report**.
- Click on **Go to Nurses' Station**.
- Click on **201** at bottom of screen.
- Click on **Patient Care**.
- Select **Nurse-Client Interactions**.
- Select and view the video titled **1500: Managing Preterm Labor**. (*Note:* If this video is not available, check the virtual clock to see whether enough time has elapsed. The video cannot be viewed before its specified time.)

2. List three nursing behaviors observed during the video interaction that reflect the nurse's acceptance of Dorothy Grant.

3. Identify three self-concept issues that a nurse should clarify about himself or herself when caring for patients.

- Click on **Chart**.
- Select the chart for Room **201**.
- Select **Consultations**.
- Review the psychiatric and social work notes.

4. The information from Dorothy Grant's medical record provides considerable information about her health problems. Complete the diagnostic process chart below.

Assessment Activities	Defining Characteristics	Nursing Diagnosis
Observe patient's nonverbal behaviors	During admission seen crying and wringing hands	_____
Observe patient's self-report of situation	Reports being scared	
Ask about decisions made or test ability to problem-solve	Reports decisions are deferred to husband	
_____	States she is unable to please husband	Situational low self-esteem
_____	"I'm scared—what am I going to do?"	
Asked to describe how she feels about situation	"I feel really _____ _____"	

5. For the diagnosis of Situational Low Self-Esteem, list three interventions you would plan for Dorothy Grant and give a rationale for each.

Fill in the blanks describing aspects of evaluation of care.

6. When evaluating a plan of care, you apply knowledge of behaviors and characteristics of a healthy _____ when you review behaviors your patient displays.

7. Key indicators of a patient's self-concept can be _____ behaviors.

8. When your plan of care involved teaching Dorothy Grant about the risks and outcomes of domestic violence, you would evaluate her ability to _____ issues pertaining to domestic violence, indicating her level of _____.

LESSON # 19

Principles Applied in Care of Older Adults

⌒ **Reading Assignment:** Growth and Development (Chapter 19, pp. 543-554)
Safety (Chapter 26)

Patients: William Jefferson, Skilled Nursing Floor, Room 403
Clarence Hughes, Medical-Surgical Floor, Room 404
Pablo Rodriguez, Medical-Surgical Floor, Room 405

Objectives:

- Describe physiologic changes of aging.
- Identify common developmental tasks of older adults.
- Differentiate among dementia, delirium, and depression.
- Discuss older adult health concerns as they apply to patients in the case studies.
- Discuss safety risks as they apply to patients in the case studies.
- Apply critical thinking to the assessment of a patient's safety risks.
- Develop a plan of care for an older adult with safety risks.

The care you provide older adults is challenging because of the normal variation in their physiologic, cognitive, and psychosocial health, as well as their functional ability. Most older adults are active and functionally independent despite the prevalence of chronic disease. However, there are those older adults who suffer from cognitive deficits and disease that result in various forms of disability. Because of the normal changes of aging being complicated by associated changes of chronic disease, the assessment of older adults can be difficult. As a nurse you must be able to understand the process of aging and not assume that all older adults have signs and symptoms representative of disease.

A major concern when caring for older adults is the ability to maintain a safe environment. Changes associated with aging increase patients' risk for falls and other accidents. As a nurse you are responsible to understand patients' risks for injury, anticipate their needs, and introduce preventive measures that ensure their safety and well-being.

Exercise 1

 CD-ROM Activity

 45 minutes

 In this exercise you will visit William Jefferson, a 75-year-old African-American male who has a history of early Alzheimer's disease and who is now in the skilled nursing unit following admission to the hospital for a urinary tract infection and sepsis. You may have worked with William Jefferson previously if you already completed Lesson 11.

• Sign in to work at Pacific View Regional Hospital on the Skilled Nursing Floor for Period of Care 1. (*Note:* If you are already in the virtual hospital from a previous exercise, click on **Leave the Floor** and then **Restart the Program** to get to the sign-in window.)
• From the Patient List, select William Jefferson (Room 501).
• Click on **Get Report**.
• Click on **Go to Nurses' Station**.
• Click on **Chart**.
• Select the chart for Room **501**.
• Click on and review the **Nursing Admission**.

1. List four developmental tasks that pose difficulties for William Jefferson and give a rationale for each.

2. William Jefferson takes eight different medications ordered by his physician. Polypharmacy increases his risk for adverse drug reactions. Explain what you would do to ensure William Jefferson takes his medications safely and appropriately once he returns home.

True or False. The nursing history reveals that William Jefferson has a hearing loss in the left ear. Select true or false for the following statements describing techniques to use to communicate better with the hearing-impaired. (*Study Tip:* Review pages 1078-1081 in your textbook.)

3. Always speak toward the ear affected by the hearing loss.
   a. True
   b. False

4. Check the ear canal for cerumen impaction.
   a. True
   b. False

5. Speak in a clear, high-pitched tone at a higher volume.
   a. True
   b. False

6. Reduce background noise during a discussion.
   a. True
   b. False

7. Encourage patients to wear their hearing devices during a conversation.
   a. True
   b. False

 • Now select and review the **History and Physical**.

8. The record indicates that William Jefferson has experienced delirium.

   a. What was the most likely cause for William Jefferson to have developed delirium?

   b. What other factors might have contributed to the delirium?

   c. How does delirium differ from dementia in regard to the following?

   Onset

   Progression

Orientation

Memory

d. Patients with Alzheimer's disease frequently also suffer depression. Depression can be distinguished from both dementia and delusions in what ways?

9. Nursing assessment of a patient with dementia and delirium is especially complex when an aging patient also suffers from chronic disease. Critical thinking applied to assessment enables a nurse to identify relevant nursing diagnoses. Complete the following critical thinking diagram for assessment of William Jefferson by writing the letter of each critical thinking factor under its proper category.

Knowledge

1. _____

2. _____

3. _____

Experience

4. _____

ASSESSMENT WILLIAM JEFFERSON

Standards

5. _____

6. _____

Attitudes

7. _____

8. _____

Critical Thinking Factors

a. Ask the patient's wife to describe how his sleep is affected when he becomes anxious or fearful.
b. Consider the effects diabetes has on physical assessment findings for vascular and neurologic function.
c. Reflect on previous encounters when you have assessed confused patients.
d. Introduce yourself when you begin to assess William Jefferson and use a calm, steady approach, explaining each step with conviction.

e. Refer to a gerontology text on the characteristics of dementia.

f. Take time in assessing William Jefferson, do not rush, and examine all body systems thoroughly.

g. Consider the effects William Jefferson's medications have on physical findings.

h. When assessing his level of discomfort, always use a pain scale.

 • Click on **Return to Nurses' Station**.

• Select Room **501** at the bottom of the screen.

• Review the **Initial Observations**.

• Click on **Patient Care**.

• Click on **Nurse-Client Interactions**.

• Select and view the video titled **0730: Intervention—Safety**. (*Note:* If this video is not available, check the virtual clock to see whether enough time has elapsed. The video cannot be viewed before its specified time.)

10. William Jefferson presents several risk factors for falls. Complete the following fall assessment tool for this patient by placing an X next to each of the clinical factors that apply to him.

_____ a. History of falls

_____ b. Confusion

_____ c. Age (over 65)

_____ d. Impaired judgment

_____ e. Sensory deficit

_____ f. Unable to ambulate independently

_____ g. Decreased level of cooperation

_____ h. Increased anxiety

_____ i. Incontinence

_____ j. Medications affecting blood pressure or consciousness

_____ k. Postural hypotension with dizziness

11. Based on what you know about William Jefferson's condition, complete the following care plan for the nursing diagnosis Risk for Falls. Provide a goal, two expected outcomes, and three interventions relevant to this patient's situation.

Nursing Diagnosis: Risk for Falls

Goal

Expected Outcomes

1.

2.

Interventions

1.

2.

3.

---

12. Which of the following devices would be useful in protecting William Jefferson from falling as he gets out of bed?
    a. Vail enclosed bed
    b. Jacket restraint
    c. Ambularm
    d. Full set of side rails

An optimal goal for all patients is a restraint-free environment. Fill in the blanks in questions 13 through 17 describing principles to follow in use of restraints.

13. A _____ order is required for the application of a restraint.

14. The use of restraints is associated with serious _____.

15. If a nurse restrains a patient because of aggressive behavior, a face-to-face physician assessment is needed within _____ hour.

16. Always secure a restraint with a _____ tie.

17. Once applied, a restraint should be removed at least every _____ hours.

Exercise 2

CD-ROM Activity

30 minutes

In this exercise you will visit Clarence Hughes, a 73-year-old African-American male with a several-year history of degenerative joint disease, osteoarthritis, and glaucoma. You may have worked with Clarence Hughes previously if you already completed Lesson 3.

- Sign in to work at Pacific View Regional Hospital on the Medical-Surgical Floor for Period of Care 1. (*Note:* If you are already in the virtual hospital from a previous exercise, click on **Leave the Floor** and then **Restart the Program** to get to the sign-in window.)
- From the Patient List, select Clarence Hughes (Room 404).
- Click on **Get Report**.
- Click on **Go to Nurses' Station**.
- Click on **Chart** and then on the chart for Room **404**.
- Click on and review the **History and Physical**.

1. Clarence Hughes reportedly has constipation.

   a. What normal physiologic change of aging might contribute to this problem?

   b. How might Clarence Hughes' osteoarthritis further contribute to constipation?

2. Clarence Hughes has a history of smoking. Smoking adds to the risks for respiratory problems. Place an X next to any of the following that describe normal physical changes in the respiratory system associated with aging.

   _____ a. Increased number of alveoli

   _____ b. Decreased cough reflex

   _____ c. Decreased vital capacity

   _____ d. Increased removal of mucus

   _____ e. Increased airway resistance

   _____ f. Increased risk for respiratory infections

➜ • Now review the **Nursing Admission**.

3. Chronic disease diminishes the well-being of older adults. Identify three nursing interventions focusing on prevention that would be appropriate for Clarence Hughes, based on his nursing admission data.

4. In order to encourage smoking cessation for Clarence Hughes, what type of intervention might you have to offer, for him to be willing to stop smoking?

5. After reviewing Clarence Hughes' admission data, describe how he has been able to meet each of the following developmental tasks.

Maintaining quality of life

Redefining relationships with adult children

Exercise 3

 CD-ROM Activity

 30 minutes

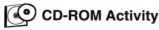 In this exercise you will visit Pablo Rodriguez, a 71-year-old Hispanic male who is suffering from advanced-stage lung cancer. You may have worked with Pablo Rodriguez previously if you already completed Lesson 6, 11, or 13.

- Sign in to work at Pacific View Regional Hospital on the Medical-Surgical Floor for Period of Care 2. (*Note:* If you are already in the virtual hospital from a previous exercise, click on **Leave the Floor** and then **Restart the Program** to get to the sign-in window.)
- From the Patient List, select Pablo Rodriguez (Room 405).
- Click on **Get Report**.
- Click on **Go to Nurses' Station**.
- Click on **Chart**.
- Select the chart for Room **405**.
- Click on and review the **Nursing Admission**.

True or False. Pablo Rodriguez admits to being "mildly depressed." Select true or false for the following statements describing features of depression.

1. Depression is typically worse in the evening hours.
   a. True
   b. False

2. A person with depression usually has reduced awareness of activities around him.
   a. True
   b. False

3. The sleep-wake cycle is usually disturbed with depression, resulting in early morning awakening.
   a. True
   b. False

4. A person who is depressed is selectively disoriented.
   a. True
   b. False

 - Click on **Return to the Nurses' Station**.
- Click on **405** to enter the patient's room.
- Review the **Initial Observations**.
- Click on **Patient Care**.
- Click on and review the assessment findings for the following categories: **Head & Neck**, **Chest**, **Upper Extremities**, and **Lower Extremities**.

5. After reviewing Pablo Rodriguez's physical findings, place an X next to any of the following findings that might be associated with a physiologic change of aging.

_____ a. Swollen gums

_____ b. Cerumen in ear canal

_____ c. Dry mouth

_____ d. Impaired chest expansion

_____ e. No adventitious sounds

_____ f. Warm skin

_____ g. Fair skin turgor

_____ h. Muscle weakness

_____ i. Swelling of leg

_____ j. Skin dry

6. What factor in Pablo Rodriguez's history would complicate these physical findings?